Advanced Nursing Series

# RESEARCH AND ITS APPLICATION

Advanced Nursing Series

# RESEARCH AND ITS APPLICATION

Edited by

## JAMES P. SMITH

*OBE, BSC (Soc), MSc, DER, SRN, RNT*
*BTA Certificate, FRCN, FRSH*

Editor of the *Journal of Advanced Nursing*
Visiting Professor of Nursing Studies
Bournemouth University

OXFORD

BLACKWELL SCIENTIFIC PUBLICATIONS

LONDON EDINBURGH BOSTON
MELBOURNE PARIS BERLIN VIENNA

This collection © 1994 by
Blackwell Scientific Publications
Editorial Offices:
Osney Mead, Oxford OX2 0EL
25 John Street, London WC1N 2BL
23 Ainslie Place, Edinburgh EH3 6AJ
238 Main Street, Cambridge,
  Massachusetts 02142, USA
54 University Street, Carlton,
  Victoria 3053, Australia

Other Editorial Offices:
Librairie Arnette SA
1, rue de Lille
75007 Paris
France

Blackwell Wissenschafts-Verlag GmbH
Düsseldorfer Str. 38
D-10707 Berlin
Germany

Blackwell MZV
Feldgasse 13
A-1238 Wien
Austria

This collection first published 1994
Full printing history of chapters can be found in
Acknowledgements

Set by DP Photosetting, Aylesbury, Bucks
Printed and bound in Great Britain by
Hartnolls Ltd, Bodmin, Cornwall.

DISTRIBUTORS
Marston Book Services Ltd
PO Box 87
Oxford OX2 0DT
(Orders: Tel: 0865 791155
          Fax: 0865 791927
          Telex: 837515)

USA
Blackwell Scientific Publications, Inc.
238 Main Street
Cambridge, MA 02142
(Orders: Tel: 800 759-6102
              617 876 7000)

Canada
Times Mirror Professional Publishing, Ltd
130 Flaska Drive
Markham, Ontario L6G 1B8
(Orders: Tel: 800 268-4178
              416 470-6739)

Australia
Blackwell Scientific Publications Pty Ltd
54 University Street
Carlton, Victoria 3053
(Orders: Tel: 03 347-5552)

British Library
Cataloguing in Publication Data
A Catalogue record for this book is available from
the British Library

ISBN 0–632–03867–5

Library of Congress
Cataloging in Publication Data
Research and its application/edited by James P.
  Smith.
      p.  cm.—(Advanced nursing series)
    Collection of updated papers originally
  published in the Journal of advanced nursing
  from 1989 to 1993.
    Includes bibliographical references and index.
    ISBN 0-632-03867-5
    1. Nursing.  2. Nursing—Research.
  I. Smith, James P., RNT.  II. Journal of
  advanced nursing.  III. Series.
    [DNLM: 1. Nursing Research—collected
  works.  WY 20.5 R4311 1994]
  RT63.R47  1994
  610.73—dc20
  DNLM/DLC
  for Library of Congress                    94-2693
                                                CIP

# Contents

# List of contributors

**Elisabeth Arborelius**, *PhD*
Assistant Professor, Department of Community Medicine, Linköping University, Linköping, Sweden.

**Karen I. Chalmers**, *RN, BScN, MSc (A), PhD*
Associate Professor, Faculty of Nursing, University of Manitoba, Winnipeg, Manitoba, Canada.

**Anna-Christina Ek**, *RN, BSc, DMSc*
Associate Professor, Department of Caring Sciences, Faculty of Health Sciences, Linköping University, Linköping, Sweden.

**Risto Erkkola**, *MD, MScD*
Acting Associate Professor, Obstetrician, Department of Obstetrics and Gynaecology, University of Turku, Turku, Finland.

**Grace Getty**, *RN, BN, MN*
Associate Professor, Faculty of Nursing, Co-ordinator of UNB Peer Education Sexual Health Program, University of New Brunswick, Fredericton, Canada.

**Taiko Hirose**, *RN, MS*
Doctoral student, School of Nursing, University of Washington, USA.

**Lennart Jorfeldt**, *MD, PhD*
Professor, Health Care Research, Department of Clinical Physiology, Linköping University, Linköping, Sweden.

**Lynda Law Harrison**, *RN, PhD*
Professor and Director of Research, The University of Alabama Capstone College of Nursing, Tuscaloosa, Alabama, USA.

**James D. Leeper**, *PhD*
Professor and Chair, Department of Behavioral and Community Medicine, The University of Alabama College of Community Health Sciences, Tuscaloosa, Alabama, USA.

**Anna Lundgren**, *RN, BA*
Lecturer, College of the Health Professions, Department of Caring Sciences, Linköping University, Linköping, Sweden.

**Edith Nonhlanhla Madela**, *RN, MCur*
DCur (Psychiatric Nursing) Candidate, Rand Afrikaans University, Johannesburg, Transvaal, Republic of South Africa.

**S. Dianne Pelletier**, *RN, BScN (Can), DipEdNsg (Sydney), BEdStudies (Qld), MSciSoc (NSW)*
Senior Lecturer, Center for Graduate Nursing Studies, University of Technology, Sydney, New South Wales, Australia.

**Marie Poggenpoel**, *RN, DPhil*
Professor of Nursing, Department of Nursing Science, Rand Afrikaans University, Johannesburg, Transvaal, Republic of South Africa.

**Päivi Rautava**, *MD, MScD*
Acting Associate Professor, Specialist in Health Care, Paediatrician, Department of Public Health, University of Turku, Turku, Finland.

**Matti Sillanpää**, *MD, MScD*
Professor, Paediatrician, Specialist in Child Neurology, Department of Child Neurology, University of Turku, Turku, Finland.

**James P Smith**, *OBE, BSc (Soc), MSc, DER, SRN, RNT, BTA Certificate, FRCN, FRSH*
Editor of the *Journal of Advanced Nursing*, and Visiting Professor of Nursing Studies, Bournemouth University, England.

**Phyllis Stern**, *DNSc, RN, FAAN, NAP*
Professor and Chair, Parent-Child Nursing, School of Nursing, Indiana University, Purdue University at Indianapolis, USA.

**Toomas Timpka**, *MD, PhD*
Assistant Professor, Departments of Community Medicine and Computer and Information Science, Linköping University, Linköping, Sweden.

**Christopher Tye**, *BSc (Hons), RGN, RMN*
Specialist Nurse Teacher (Accident and Emergency Nursing), Epsom and Kingston College of Nursing and Midwifery, Epsom, Surrey, England.

**Reiko Ueda**, *MA, DMS*
Professor of Human Development, University of Ibaraki, Ibaraki, Japan.

**Christine Webb**, *BA, MSc, PhD, SRN, RSCN, RNT*
Professor of Nursing, University of Manchester, Stopford Building, Oxford Road, Manchester M13 9PT, England.

**Mahnhee Yoon**
Doctoral Candidate (at the time of original publication), Department of

Management and Marketing, The University of Alabama, College of Commerce and Business Administration, Tuscaloosa, Alabama, USA

**Judith Young**, *RN, MScN*
Tutor, Faculty of Nursing, University of Toronto, 50 St George Street, Toronto, Ontario M5S 1A1, Canada.

# Introduction

JAMES P. SMITH,

*OBE, BSc (Soc), MSc, DER, SRN, RNT, BTA Certificate, FRCN, FRSH*
Editor of the *Journal of Advanced Nursing* and Visiting Professor of Nursing Studies,
Bournemouth University

## *Read critically*

This is the second volume of the Advanced Nursing Series and is devoted to research and its application. The contents are based on 12 papers which were originally published in the *Journal of Advanced Nursing*. Where appropriate, the papers have been updated by the authors for this publication. They are recent publications, having appeared in the journal during the past five years.

This volume should be of particular interest to undergraduate and post-graduate nursing students who are taking research method courses as part of their studies (and their teachers). The chapters are all written by aspiring and accomplished researchers so they will be of particular use to students who themselves are hoping to become involved in research activities in practice areas of nursing, midwifery and health visiting. I also hope that the book will help to foster research-mindedness among the practitioners of nursing, midwifery and health visiting (and their managers). By research-mindedness, I mean the readiness to look critically at one's work and activities and to analyse the outcomes, a willingness to encourage scientific study and an ability to use research findings where appropriate, with judgement.

The chapters in this book, therefore, need to be read critically, assumptions should be challenged, methodological limitations identified, ethical implications made explicit, and the generalizability of findings assessed with care. Perhaps some attempts might be made to refute and/or replicate the studies.

That research has captured the minds of the international community of nurses, midwives and health visitors is abundantly clear from the international mix of authors who have contributed to this publication. They share details about research conducted in Australia, Canada, England, Finland, Japan, South Africa, Sweden and the USA. Their work illustrates the use of a selection of quantitative and qualitative research methods and tools. These include the use of a case study approach, description, observation, content analysis, questionnaire, interviews, video – and the contribution of feminist research. All their literature searches are commendable.

The findings are relevant to a variety of practice settings in which nurses, midwives and health visitors work. Settings include caring for bereaved relatives in an accident and emergency department, caring for the mental health of people in a violent society, caring for mothers, infants and children, and adults, in both high technology and long term care situations, in hospitals and in the community.

It is particularly reassuring to note the emphasis on practice, as nursing, midwifery and health visiting are practice-disciplines. I am especially happy because, in a discussion about nursing research in the 1970s (Smith, 1979), I noted that, up to the 1960s, such research as there was had tended to focus on nurses rather than nursing. Although I conceded an upsurge of research interest and activities in the 1970s, particularly among British nurses, I argued that it was still very difficult to demonstrate any direct benefits from nursing research activity on patient care. I also identified a number of problems: these included the lack of experimental and replicated studies, the dearth of research-minded nurses and the apparent lack of interest in implementing nursing research findings.

## Scientific knowledge-base

I have to acknowledge that in the 15 years or so since I wrote those words, there have been indications of change. Even though there may still be room for significant developments, I think it is fair to conclude that the position so far as nursing research is concerned has moved in a progressive direction. The contents of this book certainly give support to that view.

Nevertheless, it is still true to say, as Dr Lisbeth Hockey (1980), honorary reader in nursing research, Queen Margaret College, Edinburgh, Scotland, has stated elsewhere, that:

'The knowledge-base of nursing as a professional activity is not yet adequate for the scientific support of all activities relevant to nursing care. Research is the only way in which it can be developed and it is necessary, therefore, for research to be encouraged ... Research has the potential of showing possible improvements in the administration of nursing, the education of nurses and the direct care of patients, all of which are interrelated.'

And in another publication, Professor Rosemary Crow (1981), professor of nursing studies, University of Surrey, England, has argued that, as nursing science advances:

'so it will be the mutual relationship established between research and practice which will determine both the direction of research and the means by which it makes its contribution.'

She warns that, since nursing is a dynamic process, there can never be a straightforward application of knowledge. Nor, she adds, must it be assumed that the same knowledge will be relevant at the different stages of the process of nursing.

I also want to emphasize her stress on the key role of 'clinical judgement'. It is 'a key component in the art of nursing'. She points out that this will always determine the ultimate success with which scientific nursing knowledge underlies the practice of nursing (and midwifery and health visiting).

## Studies of mothers and neonates

The first study considered in this book is the report of a major study conducted in Finland. Whilst it is written by physicians, it demonstrates that knowledge created by members of other disciplines can be very relevant to the practice of nurses, midwives and health visitors. But it should be noted that nurses and midwives participated in the research process.

Drs Rautava and Erkkola and Professor Sillanpää set out, by means of a 'postpartum questionnaire', to assess the possible influence of the expectant mother's knowledge of childbirth on the outcome and experience of pregnancy and labour. Mothers were divided into two groups according to their basic knowledge about childbirth.

All of the findings are of particular relevance to the practice of midwives and health visitors. They conclude that low levels of childbirth knowledge are associated with mothers whose babies are more frequently small for gestational age. Low knowledge is also associated with negative experiences of delivery and a negative attitude towards future pregnancies.

The second study, by Professors Harrison and Leeper and Ms Yoon, is a study of the effects of early parental touch on 36 preterm infants' heart rates and arterial saturation levels. A descriptive exploratory design was used. The infants were patients in a neonatal intensive care unit (NICU) in a southern USA hospital. A conceptual framework for the study was derived from Roy's Adaptation Model of Nursing.

This complex study involved the use of cardiac monitors to measure the infants' heart rates, and pulse oximeters to measure the arterial oxygen saturation levels in the infants. Attempts were also made to videotape each infant during three parental visits to the NICU.

The authors conclude that preterm infants' responses to early parental touch are variable. They suggest that blanket policies that limit parental touch during the early weeks of an infant's life may not be appropriate.

## Parental involvement in the care of sick children

Tokyo, Japan, provides the setting for a follow-up study of the coping behaviours of parents with children suffering from cerebral palsy. This very interesting contribution to the book is made by Ms Hirose and Professor Ueda who devised a semi-structured interview schedule for 28 mothers and 12 fathers of adult children, whose ages ranged from 22–29. The cerebral palsy children's parents had been involved in an earlier study when their children were toddlers or just starting school.

The authors conclude that male and female parental reactions to an initial diagnosis of cerebral palsy for their child are different. Furthermore, differences are noted in their use of support networks and in their individual coping strategies. Ms Hirose and Professor Ueda also argue that studies such as theirs are necessary to develop better nursing care support for the families of children suffering from handicaps.

The care of hospitalized children is the focus of a Canadian study discussed by Ms Young. It is an historical (1935–1975) case study of developments at the Hospital for Sick Children (HSC), Ontario, Canada. She was particularly interested in assessing the impact on the care of children in hospital following the introduction of 'open' visiting and family involvement in the care of their children in hospital.

However, even though these innovations received strong backing from research findings of psychological studies, she finds that the professionals at HSC lacked the conviction that change was necessary. That state of affairs persisted for many years.

Ms Young used, as primary sources, HSC annual reports, newsletters, memoranda, regulations and medical committee minutes. Nurses and doctors and patients and parents also provided oral histories. Ms Young's work suggests that paediatric nurses at HSC and other Canadian hospitals were slow to encourage family visiting and participation. Indeed the nurses were often resistant to these changes, in spite of the psychologists' strong support for them. 'Change required a major restructuring of the social system of hospital wards. This was difficult for many nurses to accept, and impossible for some,' she concludes.

### Nursing support following accidents and violence

Are nurses more amenable to meeting the needs of bereaved families in the accident and emergency department? Mr Tye attempts to answer that question, based on the views of a non-randomized, convenience sample of 52 qualified nurses working in three accident and emergency departments in hospitals in Greater London, England. He used a self-administered, structured questionnaire, using a five point Likert-type rate scale and two open-ended questions.

Mr Tye finds that, overall, the nurses have a reasonable level of awareness but 'a variety of differing perceptions of the helpfulness of individual actions'. He also notes that over half of the respondents had not received any 'death education' at any stage of their professional development. That certainly provides food for thought for nursing educators and managers.

The aim of the South African study, reported by Ms Madela and Professor Poggenpoel, was to explore the experience of a community exposed to violence and to identify the implications (and challenge) for nursing. Their research interest is very topical because, unfortunately, violence is becoming increasingly common throughout the whole world for a variety of political, religious and territorial reasons.

Ten members of a South African township community were interviewed on tape recorders. Verbatim transcripts were later subjected to a content analysis. The authors are very honest and realistic about the practical problems associated with their research activity and methods.

Much stress is noted in the community studied. But the authors conclude that violence appears to have both negative and positive effects on its victims. They believe that their findings will be of use to nursing educators in developing psychiatric nursing curricula and to multi-disciplinary teams caring for victims of violence on psychiatric wards.

They also point out that, to date, very little research has been carried out on the experience of violence, especially work on the effects of violence on children.

## Using technology in nursing practice

Both acute and long-term care of many patients now entails the use of intravenous cannulae. Ms Lundgren and Professor Jorfeldt and Dr Ek of Sweden describe a study which sought to analyse the rituals and complications surrounding the use of intravenous cannulae on 30 surgical and 30 medical patients. The authors note that documentation in the patients' records was inadequate. Thrombophlebitis is a common complication, as well as swelling, haematoma and infection. Care and handling are unsatisfactory in over half of the cases studied. Furthermore, the results of a follow-up study indicate that complications persisted for up to 150 days in some patients. The authors spell out the implications of their findings for safe nursing practice.

Ms Pelletier from Australia shares the results of a study of the experiences of hospitalized patients on whom intravenous infusion control devices were used. These devices, she argues, are nursing's responsibility as they are, to a large extent, managed by nurses. Her study was conducted in a university hospital, a public hospital and a private hospital. It is a pity, however, that no distinction was made between the correspondents from the different hospitals. That is acknowledged and remains a future research opportunity.

Patients, Ms Pelletier finds, appear to have a high level of understanding of the purpose of the device. Some 59% identified nursing staff as the source of explanation. She also concludes that devices at the bedside do not appear to be as threatening to patients 'as may have been anticipated'. That finding demonstrates an important function of research – to explode myths. Ms Pelletier also argues that nurses should endeavour to capitalize on technology as a tool to free them to focus on the patient as 38% of the patients studied did not feel they were the focus of care.

In another Swedish study, Drs Timpka and Arborelius discuss the contribution to health care of another piece of technology – the telephone. They point out that 20 million telephone calls a year are made to receptionist nurses at health care centres in Sweden. The receptionist nurse is normally the first practitioner contacted by a person with a health problem 'normally through a telephone call'. The authors set out to study the process. The telephone consultations were recorded on video. Subsequent analyses of these enabled the authors to identify the dilemmas faced by the nurses in their work.

Duration of telephone consultations ranges from one to 10 minutes and 87 dilemma situations are noted, the greatest percentage of these being 'medical-scientific' dilemmas. The authors finally point out that research findings have to be translated into the receptionist nurses' practice. This is now being organized through a local action research project. So far, the project has resulted in the creation of a specially adapted information system.

## Searching for health needs

A prime function of the United Kingdom's health visitor is to search out health needs. But, Dr Chalmers from Canada, discovering that there was a dearth of knowledge about the health visitor's work, set out to rectify the situation. Forty-five health visitors were interviewed using semi-structured, conversational interviews. A 'qualitative design in a naturalist setting' was employed and the grounded theory approach to data collection and analysis was used.

Dr Chalmers finds that health visitors do not offer all clients the same level of service. Many factors influence this. In particular, the health visitor seems to be influenced by her conceptualization of the 'overall social worth of the client situation'. The work of the health visitor is also hampered by insufficient background knowledge and burdensome 'routine' tasks. Dr Chalmers makes a number of proposals for a more effective health visiting service but she recognizes that current changes in the health care system may limit the development of new roles for health visitors.

But success in identifying health needs will certainly be enhanced by an awareness of clients' perceptions of disease and health. Ms Getty and Professor Stern therefore set out to identify gay (homosexual) men's perceptions of and responses to AIDS in Canada. AIDS and HIV are undoubted major public health concerns worldwide and it is therefore particularly appropriate to include this chapter in the book.

Using the grounded theory method to generate a theoretical framework for their data, they collected data from three sources: interviews with 34 healthy gay men; participant observation of the nursing care of men suffering from AIDS; and field notes collected after AIDS education programmes.

The authors conclude that their study provides information to help nurses care for gay men with HIV and who develop AIDS. But the findings also demonstrate the need for nurses to support gay men to attain holistic health.

## *Feminist research*

As most nurses, midwives and health visitors are women and at least half of all potential clients and patients are women, it is more than appropriate that the concluding contribution to this publication is devoted to a consideration of feminist research. An authoritative and interesting chapter is provided by Professor Webb from England, an expert writer on the topic.

Feminist research, she points out, is not simply the study of women, nor is it enough that it is done by women. It involves 'a set of principles of inquiry: a feminist philosophy of science'. An eclectic stance is generally taken in choosing feminist research methods, she says, choosing methods more appropriate to the topic rather than claiming privileged status for any particular method. Furthermore, in Professor Webb's view, feminist research should demonstrate 'relevance' to women's concerns and interests. I hasten to add that 'relevance' might be seriously considered by all researchers in nursing, midwifery and health visiting. Professor Webb makes a number of proposals for the evaluation of feminist research.

She concludes that the way forward must be to continue to acknowledge that there are a number of paradoxes and dilemmas facing feminist researchers, but ways must be sought to resolve them consistent with a 'new paradigm for nursing research'.

## *Conclusion*

The outstanding, international nurse, Dr Virginia Henderson, senior research associate emeritus, Yale University School of Nursing, USA, has summed up the major research challenge for us all. She did this in a discussion (Henderson, 1980) about preserving the essence of nursing in a technological age. We need 'imaginative and bold nurse researchers', who, through their research will bring about radical change in the basic health care of chronically ill people and other marginalized people in society, she says.

Furthermore, Virginia Henderson argues, 'nurses might more drastically affect the quality of basic nursing, if nurses developed the habits and skills of inquiry, if they applied existing research findings, and if they thought of "theory" underlying nursing as having no circumscribed limits'.

Those words of wisdom should be engraved on the hearts and minds of all who aspire to research and practise the art and science of nursing, midwifery and health visiting.

## *References*

Crow, R. (1981) Scientific nursing research: art and science. In *Nursing Science in Nursing Practice* (ed. J.P. Smith), pp. 29–42. Butterworths, London.

Henderson, V. (1980) Preserving the essence of nursing in a technological age. *Journal of Advanced Nursing*, **5**, 245–60.

Hockey, L. (1980) Research and nursing care. In *A General Textbook of Nursing (Evelyn Pearce)*, (eds J.P. Smith & P. Downie) 20th edn, pp. 362–5. Faber & Faber, London.

Smith, J.P. (1979) Is the nursing profession really research-based? *Journal of Advanced Nursing*, **4**, 319–25.

# Chapter 1
# The outcome and experiences of first pregnancy in relation to the mother's childbirth knowledge: The Finnish Family Competence Study

PÄIVI RAUTAVA, *MD, MScD*

Acting Associate Professor, Specialist in Health Care, Paediatrician, Department of Public Health

RISTO ERKKOLA, *MD, MScD*

Acting Associate Professor, Obstetrician, Department of Obstetrics and Gynaecology

and MATTI SILLANPÄÄ, *MD, MScD*

Professor, Pediatrician, Specialist in Child Neurology, Department of Child Neurology, University of Turku, Turku, Finland

The possible influence of the expectant mother's knowledge of childbirth on the outcome and experience of pregnancy and labour was investigated by means of a postpartum questionnaire in 1238 primiparae. The mothers were divided into two groups according to their basic childbirth knowledge. At birth, the conditions of newborns were equal in both groups when judged by Apgar scores. The low knowledge level group had small-for-gestational-age babies more frequently and these babies were also treated in the paediatric ward more frequently than those in the high knowledge group. The latter group was significantly more critical towards the staff of the delivery room and the postnatal ward; the fathers of this group were also present at delivery significantly more frequently. The low knowledge level group was significantly more unwilling to have another pregnancy in the near future or ever. The results indicate that low childbirth knowledge is associated with a poorer pregnancy outcome. It is a message to antenatal care staff of the need for support, supplementary education and careful obstetric surveillance. Low childbirth knowledge may imply a set of problems, including those in interparental relationship, socio-economic situation and need for close surveillance and improved education.

*Introduction*

The mother's ability to establish a good personal relationship, to stimulate her infant and to develop a rich dialogue is related to her experiences of pregnancy. A mother who wants to be pregnant accepts this condition and views motherhood positively, is better equipped to cope with pregnancy and to satisfy her infant's emotional needs (Lagercrantz, 1979; Robinson & Stewart, 1989) whereas a mother whose attitude to her pregnancy is negative will often have a similarly negative attitude to her newborn (Engström *et al.*, 1964; Trad, 1991). Interaction and co-operation with staff at the delivery hospital is important for the childbirth experience and even for acceptance of the baby (Newton & Newton, 1962; Danziger, 1979; Beaton, 1990).

Knowledge and experience greatly determine the behaviour of a human being. Health education given by the maternity health care clinic (MHCC) has traditionally aimed at increasing pregnant women's knowledge of childbearing, enabling them to make the right choices regarding health behaviour.

This study was designed to investigate whether primiparae with a greater basic knowledge of childbearing have a more positive attitude to delivery and whether any differences occur in pregnancy outcome between them and primiparae with a lower basic childbirth knowledge.

*Study population and methods*

The population of the present study was collected from the Province of Turku and Pori, south-western Finland, by means of stratified randomized cluster sampling. This represented a sample of the whole population in the province, consisting of all nulliparous women in the study area who paid their first visit to the MHCC on their own initiative during 1986.

The antenatal check-up before the 16th week of pregnancy is a prerequisite to establish eligibility for maternity benefit. Practically all pregnant women use this service which is provided free of charge. The randomization of health authority areas was carried out by drawing lots; 11 areas weighted according to their degree of urbanization were included (*Statistical Yearbook of Finland*, 1987).

Public health nurses or midwives in 67 MHCCs suggested participation to 1582 mothers, 1443 (91.2%) of whom gave their informed consent, while the remaining 139 (8.8%) refused to participate. The occupational distribution of the 139 refusers was similar to that of the participants (chi-square 3.918, d.f.s. 3, $P = 0.2705$). Other characteristics of the non-participants were not recorded (Rautava & Sillanpää, 1989).

## Data collection

Data were collected with questionnaires. The questionnaires were prepared and pretested in 1985. They were revised according to the experiences of the pilot study.

At their first visit to the MHCC (on average at the tenth week of pregnancy), the mothers completed and returned a knowledge-level questionnaire. Of the 1443 mothers, 1425 (98.9%) returned an adequately completed questionnaire. Nurses gave the mothers another questionnaire to be completed at home with questions about sociodemographic factors, health behaviour, social relations and way of life from childhood to the present pregnancy. Mothers returned the questionnaire in a closed envelope at their following visit to the clinic.

Childbirth events were enquired about in a questionnaire which the nurses gave the mothers during the home visit after the delivery (when the baby was 7–19 days old). The questionnaire consisted of questions about:

(1) Participation of the father in antenatal education and delivery, the father taking paternity leave and his attitudes towards the new family situation.
(2) Mother's experience of admission to the delivery hospital, of events in the delivery room, experiences of the first mother–infant contact, events in the postnatal ward and attitudes to future pregnancy.

Mothers returned this questionnaire in a closed envelope about 2–6 weeks later during a postpartum examination or a visit to the well-baby clinic; 1238 questionnaires were returned. The nurses completed their own questionnaires about the delivery events and newborn outcome measures according to the results of the examination during the last visit to the MHCC before delivery, and according to information obtained from the delivery hospital and during home visits. The nurses returned 1294 questionnaires.

## Statistical analysis

For statistical analysis, the mothers were divided into two groups according to their knowledge levels, with the median of correct answers as a cut-off point. The groups were designated the lower knowledge level group (LG) and the higher knowledge level group (HG).

Univariate associations with knowledge levels and childbirth events were examined using Pearson's chi-square test with Yates' correction and Mann–Whitney test when appropriate. Statistically significant variables were further examined by stepwise logistic regression analysis. The statistical analyses were carried out by means of BMDP statistical software (Dixon, 1988; Kleinbaum *et al.*, 1982).

The study design was approved by the Ethical Committee, Faculty of Medicine, University of Turku.

**Characteristics of the study population**

The mean age of the mothers was 25.4 (SD 4.3) years, range 16–42 years. At the time of their first visit to the MHCC, there were 763 married mothers (53.3%, $n = 1432$), 633 (44.2%) living in a marriage-like relationship, the remaining 36 (2.5%) were single and living alone or with their parents. Ninety-nine per cent of mothers had completed at least 9 years of primary school, and of them 42% had also finished secondary school (12 years of education). A total of 81.8% ($n = 1267$) were doing paid work (Rautava, 1989).

## *Results*

**Pregnancy course and outcome**

*Physical health during last weeks before delivery*

Maternal weight increase between the first and last weight measurements in the MHCC was 12.5 kg on average in both groups, but the LG had more mothers with a weight increase exceeding one standard deviation (16 kg) (20.0% vs. 14.4%, $P = 0.02$).

No significant differences were seen in blood pressure and use of anti-hypertensive drugs, but the LG had proteinuria more frequently (15.4% vs. 10.6%, $P = 0.02$).

No significant differences were seen in the frequency of trauma or injury between the groups, but LG had slightly more infections. LG mothers spent more time than HG mothers on sick leave immediately before maternity leave (11.6 days vs. 8.5 days, $P = 0.04$).

*Childbirth events*

HG mothers chose the university hospital as their place of delivery slightly more frequently than LG mothers, and HG mothers had slightly more operative deliveries, although these differences were not statistically significant. Caesarean section was done in 20.2%, vacuum extraction in 10.0% and forceps delivery in 2.7% of the total study population. No statistical differences were seen between the groups in the duration of pregnancy (mean 39.3 weeks and median 40.0 weeks) or the duration of delivery (LG 8.7 hours and HG 9.2 hours). The average hospital stay was eight days.

*Condition of the newborn baby*

No significant differences occurred between Apgar scores, numbers of low birthweight babies (49 babies of 2500 g or less, 3.9%) or numbers of babies delivered at less than 37 weeks of pregnancy (69 babies, 5.4%).

The average birthweight of babies was 58 g lower in the LG than in the HG. The difference was significant (3483 g vs. 3541 g, $P = 0.04$). The LG had more small-for-gestational-age babies (SGA) (13.0% vs. 7.7%, $P = 0.002$) and LG babies were treated in the paediatric ward more frequently than HG babies (57 vs. 28, $P = 0.003$).

### *In the postnatal ward*

LG babies were treated for jaundice more frequently than HG babies (64 vs. 43, $P = 0.04$). Nine per cent of all babies were given phototherapy. No difference was seen in the frequency of postnatal infections or breast inflammations.

Variables which showed statistically significant differences were further examined by stepwise logistic regression analysis. These variables were: having an SGA baby, paediatric ward care, lower birthweight, mother's weight increase during pregnancy, proteinuria, infections during pregnancy, and baby's treatment for hyperbilirubinaemia. Table 1.1 shows the final independent relations of low knowledge level to pregnancy course and outcome in stepwise logistic regression analysis.

**Table 1.1**  Pregnancy course and outcome in relation to low childbirth knowledge.

| Pregnancy course and outcome | Chi-square test in univariate analysis *P* | Stepwise logistic regression *P* | Odds ratio | 95% CI |
|---|---|---|---|---|
| SGA (small for gestational age) | 0.002 | 0.001 | | |
| No | | | 1.0 | |
| Yes | | | 2.0 | 1.4–3.0 |
| Paediatric ward care | 0.003 | 0.004 | | |
| No | | | 1.0 | |
| Yes | | | 2.0 | 1.2–3.3 |
| Lower birthweight | 0.04 | NS | | |
| Mother's weight increase (kg) | 0.02 | 0.014 | | |
| 6–16 | | | 1.0 | |
| > 20 | | | 1.5 | 0.8–2.8 |
| 16.1–20 | | | 1.6 | 1.1–2.3 |
| < 6 | | | 1.7 | 0.9–3.1 |
| Proteinuria | 0.02 | NS | | |
| Infections during pregnancy | 0.02 | NS | | |
| Treatment for hyperbilirubinaemia | 0.04 | NS | | |

**Childbirth experiences**

*Experiences of delivery hospital admission*

The HG had a more positive impression of hospital admission than the LG: they felt more frequently that the staff had been encouraging (176 vs. 144, $P = 0.03$), reassuring (397 vs. 368, $P = 0.04$) and objective (399 vs. 331, $P = 0.0001$).

*Events in the delivery room*

The LG considered the delivery room more pleasant than the HG (63 vs. 39, $P = 0.03$). The HG were more critical and found more shortcomings than the LG (75 vs. 47, $P = 0.005$). A gynaecologist took part more frequently in the delivery of HG mothers (327 vs. 252, $P = 0.0001$). HG mothers also commented on the doctor's behaviour more frequently (51 vs. 15, $P = 0.005$), pointing out that the doctor had not explained well enough about labour and delivery.

*Labour pains*

No significant difference was observed in labour pain relief or in the frequency of subjective intolerable pain between the knowledge groups. No analgesics were given to 21% of mothers, epidural anaesthesia was administered to 33% of mothers and the remainder were given injections, tablets, nitrous oxide and/or paracervical block. During labour, 35% of the mothers reported intolerable pain and 51% felt tiredness and weakness.

*Mother–infant contact*

Seventy-seven per cent of mothers were allowed to hold their babies immediately after delivery. No difference was observed in the mothers' estimation of the baby's initial success in fixing at the breast. HG mothers talked slightly more frequently to their babies during the first contact than LG mothers (518 vs. 508, $P = 0.04$).

*Experiences in the puerperal ward*

LG mothers had more difficulties in breast feeding than HG mothers (247 vs. 200, $P = 0.02$). Of all mothers, 97% breast fed their infants. More members of the HG group felt that staff were overbearing (59 vs. 33, $P = 0.005$) and commented on their performance more frequently and more critically (124 vs. 67, $P < 0.0001$) than the LG group. Almost all mothers (94%) had their baby rooming in during the hospital stay. At discharge from the delivery hospital, a paediatrician examined every baby, and the mother had an opportunity to ask questions. HG mothers asked questions significantly more often than LG mothers (351 vs. 278, $P < 0.0001$).

*Involvement of the father*

LG fathers participated in antenatal education less frequently than HG fathers (390 vs. 451, $P < 0.0001$), and they were also less frequently present at delivery (348 vs. 413, $P < 0.0001$). LG fathers were not present during the nurse's home visit as frequently as HG fathers (341 vs. 381, $P = 0.007$) and they were less frequently on paternity leave (246 vs. 300, $P = 0.0002$). The nurses estimated that HG fathers had a more positive attitude to the new family situation than LG fathers had (307 vs. 265, $P = 0.007$). The nurses did not know the mothers' knowledge groups.

*Attitude to possible and next delivery*

LG mothers wanted to have their next child only after several years. A higher number of HG mothers wanted to have another child soon (317 vs. 240, $P < 0.0001$). Of all mothers, 7.8% thought that one child was enough.

Statistically significant differences in childbirth experiences were observed in the participation of fathers (in antenatal education, delivery, at nurse's home visit and paternity leave), and fathers' attitudes to a new family situation, mothers' experiences of reception at delivery hospital, experiences of the delivery room staff, labour pains, mother–infant contact, experiences in the puerperal ward and attitudes to future pregnancy. Table 1.2 shows the final relations between low knowledge level and childbirth experiences in stepwise logistic regression analysis.

## Discussion

Birthweight distribution has proved to be a more sensitive index of environmental effects, socio-eonomic status and even antenatal socio-emotional events of the mother than miscarriages, malformations or prenatal deaths (Lewis *et al.*, 1973; Miller *et al.*, 1976; Adelstein & Fedrick, 1978; Eisner *et al.*, 1979; Ounsted & Scott, 1982; Newton & Hunt, 1984; Ericson *et al.*, 1984; Elbourne *et al.*, 1986; Ericson *et al.*, 1987; Gould & LeRoy, 1988). High, but not extreme, birthweights may also reflect positive aspects of health (Lewis *et al.*, 1973). Our LG mothers had small-for-gestational-age infants at term more frequently and the birthweights of their newborns were lower. This might indicate that a low basic childbirth knowledge in early pregnancy is

**Table 1.2**   Strongest relations of low knowledge level to pregnancy course and outcome (stepwise logistic regression analysis).

| Experiences of pregnancy | Stepwise logistic regression P | Odds ratio | 95% CI |
|---|---|---|---|
| *Participation of father* | | | |
| Took part in antenatal education | | | |
| Yes | | 1.0 | |
| No | < 0.0001 | 1.6 | 1.1–2.2 |
| On paternity leave | | | |
| Yes | | 1.0 | |
| No | 0.003 | 1.5 | 1.1–2.0 |
| *Admission at delivery hospital* | | | |
| Objective | | | |
| Yes | | 1.0 | |
| No | 0.002 | 1.5 | 1.1–2.0 |
| *Delivery room* | | | |
| Pleasant staff | | | |
| Yes | | 1.0 | |
| No | 0.010 | 1.9 | 1.2–6.1 |
| Gynaecologist at delivery | | | |
| Yes | | 1.0 | |
| No | 0.012 | 1.4 | 1.1–1.9 |
| Critical toward events | | | |
| Yes | | 1.0 | |
| No | 0.017 | 1.7 | 1.1–2.7 |
| *Puerperal ward* | | | |
| Criticizing staff | | | |
| Yes | | 1.0 | |
| No | 0.0001 | 1.8 | 1.2–2.6 |
| Asking doctor questions about the baby | | | |
| Yes | | 1.0 | |
| No | < 0.0001 | 1.6 | 1.2–2.1 |
| *Attitude to future pregnancy* | | | |
| Soon | | 1.0 | |
| Never or not for several years | < 0.011 | 1.5 | 1.1–2.0 |

associated with risks which can be eliminated with health education and social support as well as careful obstetric follow-up.

## Effectiveness of care

The absence of significant differences in the perinatal health of the newborns indicates the effectiveness of the obstetric care systems. Experts take care of the safety of labour and delivery, but although this approach guarantees high-quality management it does not necessarily guarantee positive experiences by mothers (Danziger, 1979).

In the present study, LG mothers were open-minded and submitted themselves to the care of professionals without resistance. However, their childbirth experience disappointed and even shocked them and, as a result, they became reluctant to have another baby for years to come. HG mothers, on the other hand, presented with more self-confidence, and afterwards commented critically on their experiences during labour, saying that they were ready to have another baby soon. Astbury (1980) found that antenatal education increased the knowledge of the reproductive process, but did not decrease experience of labour pain. On the other hand, Crowe & von Baeyer (1989) noticed that mothers with great knowledge of childbirth reported a less painful childbirth.

In our study, no differences occurred in the experience of labour pain, but HG mothers coped better with delivery and their attitudes to delivery were more positive afterwards than those of LG mothers. After delivery, HG mothers experienced a sense of success and tried to contact their newborn baby more eagerly. They were more inclined to feel that their breast feeding was successful than LG mothers. Davies (1988) stated in her article on breast feeding and postnatal care that the success of a mother in coping with the postnatal period will depend, to a certain extent, on the outcome of her labour, her self-perception, and the fulfilment of her expectations of the labour experience.

## Conclusions

Low childbirth knowledge, measured through a questionnaire at the first visit to the maternity health care clinic, was associated with a group of mothers whose babies were more frequently small for gestational age than those of the high knowledge group.

Low knowledge was also associated with negative delivery experiences and a negative attitude to future pregnancies. Negative experiences and events do not relate directly to low childbirth knowledge. However, a brief knowledge level questionnaire administered by public health personnel could be valuable for identification of those mothers who urgently need additional health education, social support and careful obstetric surveillance.

### Acknowledgements

The authors are grateful to those general practitioners, obstetricians, nurses and midwives who helped to collect the data and gave their invaluable comments. They wish to thank Juhani Tuominen, LicPolSc, lecturer in biostatics, Turku University Faculty of Medicine, and Olli Kaleva, MSc, who carried out the statistical analyses. Thanks are also due to Simo Merne,

MA, School of Translation Studies, University of Turku, who checked the English manuscript, and to Mrs Inger Vaihinen and Miss Eija Suopajärvi for secretarial help.

The study was financed by the Finnish National Board of Health.

## References

Adelstein, P. & Fedrick, J. (1978) Antenatal identification of women at increased risk of being delivered of a low birth weight infant at term. *British Journal of Obstetrics and Gynaecology*, **85**, 8–11.

Astbury, J. (1980) Labour pain: the role of child birth education, information and expectation. In *Problems in Pain* (eds C. Peck & M. Wallace), pp. 245–52. Pergamon, London.

Beaton, J.I. (1990) Dimensions of nurse and patient roles in labor. *Health Care for Women International*, **11**, 393–408.

Crowe, K. & von Baeyer, C. (1989) Predictors of a positive childbirth experience. *Birth*, **16**, 59–63.

Danziger, S.K. (1979) Treatment of women in childbirth: implications for family beginnings. *American Journal of Public Health*, **69**, 895–901.

Davies, R. (1988) Postnatal care and breast feeding. *Practitioner*, **232**, 1271–5.

Dixon, W.J. (ed.) (1988) *BMDP Statistical Software Manual*, vols I and II. University of California Press, Berkeley, California.

Eisner, V., Brazie, J.V., Pratt, M.W. & Hexter, A.C. (1979) The risk of low birthweight. *American Journal of Public Health*, **69**, 887–93.

Elbourne, D., Pritchard, C. & Daunce, M. (1986) Perinatal outcomes and related factors: social class differences within and between geographical areas. *Journal of Epidemiology and Community Health*, **40**, 301–8.

Engström, L., Geijerstam, G., Holmberg, N.G. & Uhrus, K. (1964) A prospective study of the relationship between psychosocial factors and course of pregnancy and delivery. *Journal of Psychosomatic Research*, **8**, 151–5.

Ericson, A., Eriksson, M., Westerholm, P. & Zetterström, R. (1984) Pregnancy outcome and social indicators in Sweden. *Acta Paediatrica Scandinavica*, **73**, 69–74.

Ericson, A., Eriksson, M., Källén, B. & Meirik, O. (1987) Birth weight distribution as an indicator of environmental effects on fetal development. *Scandinavian Journal of Social Medicine*, **15**, 11–17.

Gould, J., & LeRoy, S. (1988) Socioeconomic status and low birth weight: a racial comparison. *Pediatrics*, **82**, 896–904.

Kleinbaum, D.G., Kupper, L.L. & Morgenstern, H. (1982) *Epidemiologic Research*. Lifetime Learning Publication, Belmont, California.

Lagercrantz, E. (1979) *Primiparas and their infants*. A psychological study of pregnancy, delivery and motherhood during the infant's first eighteen months of life and of the infant's development. (English summary). Doctoral thesis, Karolinska Institutet, Stockholm.

Lewis, R., Charles, M. & Patwary, K.M. (1973) Relationship between birthweight and selected social, environmental and medical care factors. *American Journal of Public Health*, **63**, 973–81.

Miller, H.C., Hassanein, K., Chin, T.D.Y. & Hensleigh. (1976) Socioeconomic factors in relation to fetal growth in white infants. *Journal of Pediatrics*, **89**, 638–43.

Newton, N. & Newton, M. (1962) Mothers' reactions to their newborn babies. *Journal of the American Medical Association*, **181**, 206–10.

Newton, R.W. & Hunt, L.P. (1984) Psychosocial stress in pregnancy and its relation to low birth weight. *British Medical Journal*, **288**, 1191–4.

Ounsted, M. & Scott, A. (1982) Social class and birthweight: a new look. *Early Human Development*, **6**, 83–9.

Rautava, P. (1989) The Finnish Family Competence Study: characteristics of pregnant women with low childbirth knowledge. *Social Science and Medicine*, **29**, 1105–9.

Rautava, P. & Sillanpää, M. (1989) Knowledge of childbirth of nulliparae seen at maternity health care clinics. *Journal of Epidemiology and Community Health*, **43**, 253–60.

Robinson, G.E. & Stewart, D.E. (1989) Motivation for motherhood and experience of pregnancy. *Canadian Journal of Psychiatry*, **34**, 861–5.

*Statistical Yearbook of Finland* (1987) vol. 82. Central Statistical Office of Finland, Helsinki.

Trad, P.V. (1991) Adaptation to developmental transformations during the various phases of motherhood. *Journal of the American Academy of Psychoanalysis*, **19**, 403–21.

# Chapter 2
# Effects of early parent touch on preterm infants' heart rates and arterial oxygen saturation levels

LYNDA LAW HARRISON, *RN, PhD*
Professor and Director of Research, The University of Alabama Capstone College of Nursing

JAMES D. LEEPER, *PhD*
Professor and Chair, Department of Behavioral and Community Medicine, The University of Alabama College of Community Health Sciences

and MAHNHEE YOON
Doctoral Candidate (at the time of original publication), Department of Management and Marketing, The University of Alabama, College of Commerce and Business Administration, Tuscaloosa, Alabama, USA

A descriptive exploratory design was used in this study to evaluate the effects of early parent touch on the heart rates and arterial oxygen ($O_2$) saturation levels of 36 preterm infants. The infants were between 27 and 33 weeks gestational age at birth, and were free of congenital defects. Infants were videotaped during parent visits on up to three separate occasions during the first month of life. Parents were encouraged to interact with their infants as they usually would, and data on the infants' heart rates and $O_2$ saturation levels were recorded every six seconds on a portable computer that was interfaced with the infants' monitors. Mean $O_2$ saturation levels were significantly lower during parent touch than during baseline periods on 45% of the visits, and significantly higher during parent touch periods on 19% of the visits. $O_2$ saturation variability was greater during periods of parent touch, and there were more abnormal $O_2$ saturation values during parent touch than during baseline periods. Mean heart rates during parent touch were significantly lower compared to baseline on 17% of the visits, and were higher during parent touch on 43% of the visits. There were no overall differences in mean heart rates between baseline, parent touch and post-visit classifications, although heart rate variability was greater during periods of parent touch. The results indicate that preterm infants' responses to early parent touch are variable, and suggest that blanket policies that limit parent touch during the early weeks of life may not be appropriate. It may be more appropriate to teach parents to modify the types and amounts of touch they provide based on the infants' physiologic and behavioural cues.

## Introduction

Although touch may be an important mediator of the development of attachment between parents and infants, nurses often discourage parents from touching their preterm infants because of the infant's compromised health status and the hypoxia which can result from excessive handling (Miller & Holditch-Davis, 1992). Yet many parents have noted that early opportunities for tactile contact with their preterm infants help them to cope with their feelings of loss, and to begin to develop feelings of closeness towards their infants (Nance, 1982). The question of whether early parent touch has adverse effects on preterm infants has not yet been answered. The purpose of this study was to describe the effects of early parent touch on the heart rates and arterial oxygen saturation levels of preterm infants during the first two to four weeks of the infants' lives.

## Conceptual framework

Touch is the 'earliest and most elemental medium of human communication' (Barnett, 1972). Appropriate tactile experience is essential for the optimal growth and development of the infant, and for the development of parent–infant attachment (Frank, 1957; Harlow, 1958; Klaus & Kennell, 1982). The study was based on a conceptual framework for analysing the meaning of touch that was developed by Weiss (1979).

Roy's (1984) adaptation model provided the nursing conceptual framework for this study. This model incorporates concepts from adaptation and systems theory. The focus of nursing may be individuals or groups which are viewed as open systems. In this study, the preterm infant was the system of interest. Roy (1984) identified three types of stimuli that comprise system inputs: (a) focal stimuli (those immediately confronting the person); (b) contextual stimuli (all other internal and external stimuli); and (c) residual stimuli (values, beliefs, traits or attitudes which may influence the system). The system output is conceptualized by Roy as either adaptive (promoting the integrity of the system), or maladaptive (failing to promote system growth). The goal of nursing is to enhance stimuli that lead to adaptive responses and modify stimuli that lead to maladaptive responses. This study examined the effects of a specific focal stimulus (parental touch) on the immediate physiological adaptation of preterm infants.

This research was part of a larger project that was also designed to describe the physical characteristics of touch used by parents in touching their preterm infants, and to determine whether infants' physiological responses to parent touch were affected by certain contextual stimuli (such as a gestational age or morbidity status). Other results from the larger study are reported elsewhere (Harrison, 1989a).

## Related literature

There has been relatively little research to describe preterm infants' sensitivities to different types of tactile stimuli. Haith (1986) noted that all body parts are sensitive to cutaneous stimuli by 32 weeks gestational age, although Rose *et al.* (1976) found that preterm infants (with a mean gestational age of 33.2 weeks) showed minimal behavioural responses and no significant cardiac responses to abdominal tactile stimulation with a plastic filament.

Few studies were found that focused on the infants' immediate physiological or behavioural responses to tactile stimulation. Beaver (1987) evaluated the effects of supplemental stroking during a heel stick procedure on eight preterm infants who were between 32 and 34 weeks gestational age at birth. Each infant received three treatments in a random order: (a) heel touch only; (b) heel stick; or (c) stroking the leg while a heel stick was performed. The third treatment (stroking during the heel stick) resulted in the greatest change in all three physiologic parameters, with increases in blood pressure and heart rate, and a decrease in transcutaneous oxygen ($T_cPO_2$) levels.

White-Traut & Goldman, (1988) found that preterm infants' heart and respiratory rates increased following a multimodal stimulation treatment that included tactile, visual, auditory and vestibular stimulation. Although the physiologic parameters stabilized 20 minutes following the treatment, the researchers concluded that preterm infants' immediate responses to stimulation regimens should be monitored closely.

Peters (1992) assessed responses of ten preterm infants to various types of medical and nursing procedures that involved handling. Infants experienced 120–245 contacts during a 24-hour period. Even procedures associated with minimal handling (such as auscultating heart rates) often result in hypoxia, oxygen desaturation, or increased levels of intracranial pressure.

### Stroking

Oehler (1985) examined the physiologic responses of 15 preterm infants (ranging from 26–30 weeks gestational age at birth) to tactile and auditory stimulation, and found that $T_cPO_2$ levels remained the same or increased during auditory stimulation, but tended to decrease during touching or simultaneous touching/talking. Oehler stressed the need for further research to determine whether 'ways of providing tactile stimulation other than stroking may prove to be enriching for the infants and not cause avoidance behaviors or hypoxia'.

Oehler *et al.* (1988) suggested that the adverse effects of stroking may have detrimental effects only for the less mature high-risk infants, and advocated further research to examine subgroup differences among high- and low-risk preterm infants' response to touch. Powell (1974) noted that many of the smallest babies in her study 'reacted to (the) stroking as if it were quite noxious'. This comment is particularly significant in the light of recent studies which have demonstrated that excessive handling associated with medical/nursing procedures results in hypoxaemia in very small preterm infants (Long *et al.*, 1980; Norris *et al.*, 1982; Speidel, 1978). Hypoxia and blood pressure elevations which may result from excessive handling may lead to intraventricular haemorrhage in preterm infants, particularly in those who are less than 32 weeks gestational age (Tardy & Volpe, 1982). In order to minimize the risk of hypoxia and intraventricular haemorrhage, a number of researchers and clinicians have advocated limiting the handling of very small preterm infants (Long *et al.*, 1980; Lucey, 1981; Speidel, 1978; personal communication from W.H. Tooley to L. Harrison, 19 June 1984). Luddington (1983), in proposing guidelines for stimulation of high-risk infants, suggested that prematures less than 32 weeks gestation should receive no additional tactile or vestibular stimulation during the first ten days of life.

Gorski *et al.* (1983) stressed the need for research based on direct observation of preterm infants' responses to stimuli provided in the neonatal intensive care unit (NICU). No studies were found that described, specifically, how parents touch their hospitalized preterm infants or evaluated infants' physiologic responses to parent touch. Similarly, no research was identified that compared the types of touch provided for preterm infants by parents with that provided by non-parent caregivers. Observation of preterm infants' responses to parental contact are particularly important in view of the widespread concern about promoting early parent–infant contact in order to enhance infant development and parent–infant attachment, while at the same time preventing complications (such as hypoxia) which could lead to adverse neurologic sequelae in the infants.

## Study questions

Two questions guided this study:

(1) What are the effects of parental touch on the heart rates of preterm infants?

(2) What are the effects of parental touch on the arterial oxygen saturation levels of preterm infants?

## Methods

### Subjects and setting

The subjects for this study were 36 preterm infants who were between 25 and 33 weeks gestational age at birth, and their parents. The infants were patients in an NICU in the southern United States that serves as a regional referral centre. The infants had no congenital anomalies and had not undergone surgery. Parents were told that the purpose of the study was to learn about preterm infants' responses to stimulation provided during parent visits, including tactile stimulation, and those who agreed to participate signed informed consent forms. A total of 17 parents declined to participate in the study. Of the 36 infants in the sample, 14 were male and 22 were female. Twelve infants were white and 24 were black. The mean gestational age of the infants at birth was 29.6 weeks (SD 2.4), and the mean birthweight was 1337 grams (SD 403, range 688–2080).

### Instruments and measurements

The infants' *heart rates* were measured by continuous recordings from Corametric cardiac monitors. The infants' *arterial oxygen* ($O_2$) *saturation levels* were measured by continuous recordings from a Nellcor pulse oximeter. The pulse oximeter consists of a small probe containing two light-emitting diodes and a photosemiconducter which was attached to the infant's forefoot. Deckardt & Steward (1984) reported that $O_2$ saturation levels were correlated with transcutaneous oxygen ($T_cPO_2$) levels over a wide range of $O_2$ saturations. In addition, pulse oximeter readings were closely correlated with *in vivo* arterial oxygen saturation readings. These authors suggested that the oxygenation status of hypoxaemic infants may be more sensitively measured by pulse oximeters than by $T_cPO_2$ monitors. In addition, pulse oximeters do not pose the risk of skin burns to the infants which accompanies the use of $T_cPO_2$ monitors (Deckardt & Steward, 1984). The primary source of measurement error with pulse oximetry is motion artifact in extremely active infants (New, 1985). Heat lamps, radiant warmers and phototherapy lights might also affect pulse oximetry readings. However, this problem can usually be avoided by shielding the sensor (Jennis & Peabody, 1987).

The reliability of the oximeter readings was assessed by comparing the heart rate readings on the pulse oximeter with those on the Corametric cardiac monitor in order to ensure an adequate pulsatile blood flow as suggested by Deckhardt & Steward (1984). All sensors were covered with probe covers supplied by the Nellcor Corporation. When the $O_2$ saturation levels were distorted because of motion artifact, those readings were not included in the analysis. For a more complete discussion of the procedures used to reduce the risk of measurement error in this study, see Harrison (1989b).

The infant's *gestational age* was assessed by the neonatologists in the study NICU, using the system described by Ballard *et al.* (1979).

## Procedures

A descriptive exploratory design was used to answer the study questions. Because no previous studies were found that described the specific physical characteristics of touch used by parents of preterm infants, the researchers decided not to impose controls on the types of touch to be provided. Once data are available describing the physical characteristics of early parent touch, more controlled studies can be implemented to evaluate the physiologic effects of the types of parent touch that are most often provided to preterm infants.

Attempts were made to videotape each study infant during three parent visits to the NICU when the infants were between five and 14 days of age. For some infants, the data collection times had to be altered because parents were unable to visit the NICU during the specified data collection times, or the infants' medical conditions were unstable and the physicians requested that the parents should not touch the infants. Twenty-seven infants were videotaped during three parent visits, six were taped during two visits, and three were videotaped during only one visit. The mean ages of the infants during the three visits were 5.8, 8.4 and 11.3 days, respectively.

A Compaq portable computer was interfaced with the infant's Corametric cardiac monitor and Nellcor pulse oximeter with an analog-to-digital converter (ADC). A computer program was developed using the Asyst software package to program the interface between the computer and the ADC. Data on the infant's heart rate and arterial oxygen saturation levels were recorded every six seconds by the computer, and stored on a hard disk. The researcher checked the readings on the monitors and the computer screen periodically throughout the data collection periods, to ensure that they were consistent. The videocamera was interfaced with the computer using a videocombiner, so that data on the time, observation number and the physiologic parameters were recorded on the videotape.

Physiologic parameters were recorded for a five-minute baseline period before the parents approached the infants' bedsides. Once the parents approached the bedside, the researcher adjusted the focus of the videocamera, and then left the bedside to decrease the possibility that parents might become anxious as a result of an observer's presence. Parents were encouraged to interact with their infants as they usually would, and at the end of the visits were given a copy of the videotape to keep. At the end of the parent visit, post-visit data were collected for 10 minutes. The NICU staff were aware of the study purposes and generally tried not to interrupt the parents during the visit. If, however, the infants required care during the data collection periods, the staff provided such care. It was possible to identify when the infants were touched by NICU staff (as opposed to parents) when the videotapes were coded, so that the effects of parent and nurse touch could be analysed separately.

The videotapes were subsequently coded to describe the physical characteristics of parent touch and to identify the specific observation periods during which parent or nurse touch occurred. This information was interfaced with the physiologic data files on a mainframe computer so that it was possible to compare the infants' physiologic responses during parent touch episodes. Episodes of nurse touch were not included in this analysis.

## Data analysis

As a preliminary analysis, one-way ANOVA procedures were used to analyse changes across three touch classifications (baseline, parent touch and post-visit) for each visit. It was recognized that there were not independent observations in these analyses, since infants were measured on more than one visit, and the touch classification was actually a within-subjects factor. In addition, there was variability in the number of observations in the touch classification periods, since the amount of touch provided varied among parents. However, this analysis provided information about general trends in the data. Because of the large number of observations and the possibility of a Type 1 error, a conservative alpha level of 0.001 was used for these analyses.

The mean $O_2$ saturation level during parent touch was significantly lower than baseline on 35 out of 78 visits (45%) that were analysed. The decrease in mean $O_2$ saturation during parent touch was considered clinically significant (i.e. decreasing from a value of greater than 90% to a value of less than 90%) for only 6 (8%) visits. For 15 of the 78 visits (19%), the mean $O_2$ saturation during parent touch was significantly higher than during the baseline period. For three visits (4%), the increase was considered clinically significant, changing from a mean baseline reading of less than 90% to a mean above 90% during parent touch.

Mean heart rates during parent touch were significantly lower than baseline on 14 of 84 visits (17%) for which complete heart rate data were available. The mean heart rate was significantly higher during parent touch than baseline on 36 (43%) visits. None of the heart rate means were outside of clinically acceptable ranges of 100–200 beats per minute (Fig. 2.1).

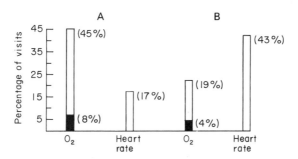

**Fig. 2.1**   Percentage of visits during which $O_2$ and heart rate levels increased or decreased from baseline to parent touch. A = mean values lower during baseline than parent touch. B = mean values higher during baseline than parent touch. ■ = clinically significant change.

Repeated measures ANOVAs were then computed using $O_2$ and heart rate means and standard deviations as dependent variables, with both touch classification (baseline, parent touch and post-visit) and visit number as the within-subjects factors. A 0.05 level of significance was used for all of the repeated measures ANOVAs. Because it was necessary to have equal numbers of observations in each group for a repeated measures ANOVA, the data for this analysis consisted of the means and standard deviations for each of the three touch classifications of each case. Cases were included in these analyses only if there were more than 10 instances (i.e. 60 seconds) of parent touch, and if there were complete data for all three visits and for both baseline and post-visit classifications.

The results of the first repeated measures ANOVA indicated that there were no differences in $O_2$ saturation across the three touch classifications, although there was a significant visit effect with the highest $O_2$ mean noted on visit 1, and the lowest noted on visit 3 (Table 2.1). There were significant effects for visit and touch classification on $O_2$ saturation standard deviation, with more variability during parent touch, and on the third visit.

The results of the second repeated measures ANOVA indicated that there were no effects on heart rate mean based on touch classification, but there were visit effects, with the mean heart rate being slightly higher on visit 3 than on visits 1 or 2 (Table 2.2). Heart rate variability was significantly higher during parent touch, although there were no visit effects for heart-rate variability.

The final step in analysing the data was to use non-parametric Friedman analysis procedures to assess the differences in ranks of abnormal $O_2$ and heart-rate values across the touch classification periods (Tables 2.3 and 2.4). For the purpose of this analysis, $O_2$ values that were less than 90% were considered abnormal, and heart-rate values that were less than 100 or more than 200 beats per minute were considered abnormal. There were more abnormal $O_2$ saturation values during parent touch than during baseline

**Table 2.1**  Results of repeated measures ANOVAs on O$_2$ saturation mean and standard deviation by touch classification and visit number.

| | O$_2$ mean | | | | | | O$_2$ standard deviation | | | | | |
| --- | --- | --- | --- | --- | --- | --- | --- | --- | --- | --- | --- | --- |
| Time | Baseline | Parent touch | Post-visit | Overall mean | P for visit | P for touch classification | Baseline | Parent touch | Post-visit | Overall mean | P for touch | P for touch classification |
| Visit 1 | 95.1 | 95.3 | 95.0 | 95.1[a] | | | 1.9 | 2.5 | 2.4 | 2.3[a] | | |
| Visit 2 | 95.3 | 93.5 | 93.7 | 94.2 | | | 2.0 | 3.5 | 3.0 | 2.8 | | |
| Visit 3 | 93.6 | 92.7 | 94.3 | 93.5[b] | | | 2.9 | 4.3 | 2.6 | 3.3[b] | | |
| Overall mean | 94.7 | 93.8 | 94.3 | | 0.05 | 0.24 | 2.3[a] | 3.4[b] | 2.7[a] | | 0.01 | 0.001 |

d.f. = 2, 32. [a] and [b] notations indicate means that were significantly different from one another.

**Table 2.2**  Results of repeated measures ANOVAs on heart rate mean and standard deviation by touch classification and visit number.

| | Heart rate mean | | | | | | Heart rate standard devision | | | | | |
| --- | --- | --- | --- | --- | --- | --- | --- | --- | --- | --- | --- | --- |
| Time | Baseline | Parent touch | Post-visit | Overall mean | P for visit | P for touch classification | Basline | Parent touch | Post-visit | Overall mean | P for visit | P for touch classification |
| Visit 1 | 145.4 | 146.4 | 147.1 | 146.3[a] | | | 5.5 | 7.1 | 5.9 | 6.2 | | |
| Visit 2 | 152.5 | 152.6 | 152.0 | 152.4 | | | 5.4 | 6.8 | 6.2 | 6.1 | | |
| Visit 3 | 154.3 | 156.4 | 152.0 | 154.2[b] | | | 7.2 | 9.0 | 7.1 | 7.8 | | |
| Overall mean | 150.7 | 151.8 | 150.4 | | 0.04 | 0.22 | 6.0[a] | 7.6[b] | 6.4[a] | | 0.20 | 0.02 |

[a] and [b] notations indicate means that were significantly different from one another.

**Table 2.3**  Means, medians, ranks and results of Friedman analyses for percentage of abnormal $O_2$ saturation values by touch classification.

| Time | Touch classification | | | Chi-square | d.f.[a] | P |
|------|---------|-------------|-----------|------------|------|---|
|      | Baseline | Parent touch | Post-visit |            |      |   |
| *Visit 1* | | | | | | |
| Mean | 17.0 | 18.5 | 22.4 | | | |
| Median | 0.9 | 5.4 | 6.9 | | | |
| Rank | 1.70 | 2.20 | 2.09 | 4.42 | 2 | 0.11 |
| Number of | | | | | | |
| cases | 32 | | | | | |
| *Visit 2* | | | | | | |
| Mean | 18.0 | 22.9 | 23.7 | | | |
| Median | 0.0 | 9.8 | 13.8 | | | |
| Rank | 1.50[a] | 2.24[b] | 2.26 | 8.63 | 2 | 0.01 |
| Number of | | | | | | |
| cases | 23 | | | | | |
| *Visit 3* | | | | | | |
| Mean | 17.6 | 31.7 | 21.1 | | | |
| Median | 10.8 | 31.3 | 4.0 | | | |
| Rank | 1.81 | 2.50[a] | 1.69[b] | 6.86 | 2 | 0.03 |
| Number of | | | | | | |
| cases | 18 | | | | | |
| *Visits 1–3 combined* | | | | | | |
| Mean | 17.4 | 23.2 | 22.5 | | | |
| Median | 0.0 | 10.7 | 7.2 | | | |
| Rank | 1.66[a] | 2.29[b] | 2.05 | 14.43 | 2 | 0.001 |
| Number of | | | | | | |
| cases | 73 | | | | | |

[a] and [b] notations indicate ranks that were significantly different from one another by applying Friedman analyses to pairs of touch classifications.

periods on all visits, and these differences were statistically significant on the second visit and when data from all three visits were combined. There were significantly more abnormal $O_2$ values during parent touch than during the post-visit period on the third visit. There were relatively few abnormal heart-rate values, and there were no significant differences in percentage of abnormal heart-rate values across the three touch classifications.

## Discussion

### Effects of parent touch on infants' $O_2$ saturation levels

There was considerably variability in the effects of parent touch on infants' haemoglobin oxygen saturation levels. Although the $O_2$ saturation levels

**Table 2.4**   Means, medians, ranks and results of Friedman analyses for percentage of abnormal heart rate values by touch classification.

| Time | Touch classification | | | Chi-square | d.f.[a] | P |
|------|----------|--------------|------------|------------|------|---|
|      | Baseline | Parent touch | Post-visit |            |      |   |
| *Visit 1* | | | | | | |
| Mean | 1.0 | 0.2 | 0.3 | | | |
| Median | 0.0 | 0.0 | 0.0 | | | |
| Rank | 1.95 | 2.11 | 1.94 | 0.58 | 2 | 0.75 |
| Number of | | | | | | |
| cases | 32 | | | | | |
| *Visit 2* | | | | | | |
| Mean | 0.2 | 0.2 | 0.5 | | | |
| Median | 0.0 | 0.0 | 0.0 | | | |
| Rank | 1.91 | 2.00 | 2.09 | 0.35 | 2 | 0.84 |
| Number of | | | | | | |
| cases | 23 | | | | | |
| *Visit 3* | | | | | | |
| Mean | 1.9 | 0.5 | 0.3 | | | |
| Median | 0.0 | 0.0 | 0.0 | | | |
| Rank | 1.97 | 2.17 | 1.86 | 0.86 | 2 | 0.65 |
| Number of | | | | | | |
| cases | 18 | | | | | |
| *Visits 1–3 combined* | | | | | | |
| Mean | 1.0 | 0.3 | 0.4 | | | |
| Median | 0.0 | 0.0 | 0.0 | | | |
| Rank | 1.95 | 2.09 | 1.97 | 0.88 | 2 | 0.64 |
| Number of | | | | | | |
| cases | 73 | | | | | |

were significantly lower during parent touch than baseline on 45% of the visits, the values were significantly higher during parent touch on 19% of the visits. The results of the Friedman analyses indicated that there were more abnormal $O_2$ saturation values during parent touch than during baseline or post-visit periods.

The results of the repeated measures ANOVAs indicated that there were no differences in $O_2$ saturation levels across the three touch classifications, although there was more variability in $O_2$ saturation levels during parent touch than during baseline and post-visit periods. These findings are consistent with the results of the one-way ANOVAs, and suggest that preterm infants do respond physiologically to parent touch, but that individual infants vary in their responses.

The mean $O_2$ saturations were slightly but significantly higher on the first visit than on the third visit, but there was significantly more variability on $O_2$ saturation during the third visit. This finding was surprising, since the medical conditions of the infants were generally less stable on the first than on subsequent visits. One explanation for this finding might be that more infants were in ventilators during the first visit. The higher and less variable $O_2$ levels during the first visit may have resulted from the supplemental oxygen that many infants were receiving.

These findings are consistent with the findings of Beaver (1987), Long *et al.* (1980), Norris *et al.* (1982), Peters (1992) and others, correlating excessive handling with an increased incidence of hypoxia in preterm infants. This study is different from the other studies in that it specifically examined the handling provided by parents during the early weeks of life. It is important to note that although the number of abnormal $O_2$ saturation levels increased during periods of parent touch, when analysing individual infant data it became apparent that some infants responded more favourably to parent touch, with increased mean $O_2$ saturation levels and a decrease in the percentage of abnormal $O_2$ saturation values. These findings suggest that NICU policies that limit all parent touch for preterm infants may not be appropriate. It may be more advisable to teach parents to modify the types and amounts of touch they provide based on the infants' behavioural and physiological responses, as suggested by Oehler (1985). Parents could be taught to observe the infant's $O_2$ saturation monitors, for example, and to alter their patterns of touching if the levels began to decrease. Likewise, they could be encouraged to continue their patterns of touching if the $O_2$ levels remained the same or increased.

### Effects of parental touch on infant heart rate

There was also considerable variability in the effects of parental touch on infant heart rate, although there were very few abnormal heart-rate values observed during any of the touch classification periods. There were significant decreases in mean heart rate during parent touch compared to baseline on 17% of the visits, and significant increases on 43% of the visits, but none of the differences in heart rate were considered clinically significant. The results of repeated measured ANOVAs indicated that there were no differences in mean heart rate across the three touch classification periods, although heart-rate variability was significantly higher during parent-touch periods. The mean heart rate was higher during the third visit.

These findings indicate that infant heart rate was less affected by parent touch than $O_2$ saturation. This finding suggests that heart rate response may be a less effective indicator of the effects of tactile stimulation on preterm infants than $O_2$ saturation. The finding of increased heart-rate variability during parent touch suggests that preterm infants do respond to tactile stimulation. Rose *et al.* (1976) found that preterm infants showed no cardiac responses to tactile stimuli provided by three different plastic filaments. It is likely that the touch provided by the parents was stronger than the stimulation provided in the Rose *et al.* (1976) study and therefore the infants in the present study demonstrated a greater cardiac response to touch.

## Recommendations for further research

The present study raised a number of questions for further research. There is a need for further analysis of the data from the present study to explain the variability in infants' physiologic responses to touch. Analyses of the effects of a number of contextual stimuli (such as gestational age, morbidity status, behavioural state and amount of handling prior to the parent visit) have been conducted by the authors (Harrison, Leeper, & Yoon, 1991).

Lower gestational age was associated with a greater percentage of abnormally low $O_2$ saturation values during parent touch. Smaller infants and those who had received more handling during the two hours prior to the parent visit had fewer abnormal heart rate values during parent touch. One explanation for this finding may be that few abnormal heart rate values were observed, and the results may have been skewed by atypical responses of a few infants.

Another factor that may have contributed to the variability in the infants' responses to touch is the different types and amounts of touch provided by the parents. Harrison and Woods (1991) examined the types of touch provided by mothers, fathers and grandmothers in the present study. The mean total duration of touch provided during the visits was 17.5 minutes. The standard deviation was 22.6 minutes (suggesting high variability in the amounts of touch provided). Parents most frequently held, stroked, or simply had tactile contact with their infants.

Because a descriptive, exploratory design was used in the present study, it was not possible to control many extraneous variables that may have influenced the infants' responses to parent touch. For example, there was variability in the types and amounts of touch the parents provided. In addition, it was not possible to completely control the handling provided by NICU staff during the parent visits, or changes in the percentage of oxygen received by the infants who were receiving supplemental oxygen. More controlled studies are needed in which the specific effects of different types of touch are examined. These studies could utilize quasi-experimental time-series designs, in which researchers provide the types of tactile stimulation most often provided by parents.

## Parents

There is also a need for more research to identify the meaning of touch to parents of preterm infants. How do parents feel about touching their small preterm infants in the NICU? Do restrictions on parent touch interfere with the development of parent–infant attachment? Do specific suggestions from the NICU staff about how to touch small preterm infants help parents feel more comfortable handling their infants? Qualitative research designs could address these questions.

Finally, research is needed to determine the effectiveness of nursing interventions that are designed to teach parents to modify the tactile stimulation they provide to their preterm infants based on the infant's physiological and behavioural responses to such stimulation.

## Acknowledgements

This research was supported by a new Investigator Award from the National Center for Nursing Research(#1R23 NU01628). The Nellcor Corporation loaned the use of a pulse oximeter for the study.

The author wishes to acknowledge the support of the NICU staff at DCH Regional Medical Center in Tuscaloosa, Alabama, and of the following consultants and research assistants: Linda Day, RN, Peter Gorski, MD, Joe Hanson, Ashley McCord, RN, Louis Sheppard, PhD, Sandra Weiss, DN, SC, and Stephanie Woods, RN, MSN. A special appreciation is extended to the parents and infants whose participation made this study possible.

## References

Ballard, J.L., Novak, K.K. & Driver, M. (1979) A simplified score for assessment of fetal maturation of newly born infants. *Journal of Pediatrics*, **95**, 769.

Barnett, K. (1972) A theoretical construct of the concepts of touch as they relate to nursing. *Nursing Research*, **21**, 102–10.

Beaver, P.K. (1987) Premature infants' response to touch and pain: can nurses make a difference? *Neonatal Network*, **6**(3), 13–17.

Deckardt, R. & Steward, D.J. (1984) Noninvasive arterial hemoglobin oxygen saturation versus transcutaneous oxygen tension monitoring in the preterm infant. *Critical Care Medicine*, **12**(11), 935–9.

Frank, L.K. (1957) Tactile communication. *Genetics Psychological Monographs*, **56**, 211–51.

Gorski, P.A., Hale, W.T., Leonard, C.H. & Martin, J.A. (1983) Direct computer recording of premature infants and nursery care: distress following two interventions. *Pediatrics*, **72**, 198–202.

Haith, M.M. (1986) Sensory and perceptual processes in early infancy. *The Journal of Pediatrics*, **109**(1), 158–71.

Harlow, H.F. (1958). The nature of love. *American Psychologist*, **13**, 673–85.

Harrison, L.L. (1989a) *Effects of early parent touch on preterm infants*. Final grant report submitted to the National Center for Nursing Research, no. NR01628-03 (now National Institute for Nursing Research), Bethesda, Maryland.

Harrison, L.L. (1989b) Interfacing bioinstruments with computers for data collection in nursing research. *Research in Nursing and Health*, **12**, 129–33.

Harrison, L.L., Leeper, J. & Yoon, M. (1991). Preterm infants' physiologic responses to early parent touch. *Western Journal of Nursing Research*, **13**, 706–21.

Harrison, L.L. & Woods, S. (1991). Early parental touch and preterm infants. *Journal of Obstetric, Gynaecologic, and Neonatal Nursing*, **20**, 299–306.

Jennis, M.S. & Peabody, J.L. (1987) Pulse oximetry: an alternative method for the assessment of oxygenation in newborn infants. *Pediatrics*, **79**(4), 524–7.

Klaus, M.H. & Kennell, J.H. (1982) *Parent–infant bonding*, 2nd edn. C.V. Mosby, St Louis.

Long, J.G., Philip, A.G.S. & Lucey, J.F. (1980) Excessive handling as a cause of hypoxemia. *Pediatrics*, **65**(2), 203–7.

Lucey, J.F. (1981) Clinical uses of transcutaneous oxygen monitoring. In *Advances in Pediatrics*, **28**, 27–55.

Luddington, S. (1983, June) *Infant stimulation: new concepts in neonatal/infant growth and development*. Workshop sponsored by Symposia Medicus, Dallas, Texas.

Miller, D.B. & Holditch-Davis, D. (1992). Interactions of parents and nurses with high-risk preterm infants. *Research in Nursing and Health*, **15** 187–97.

Nance, S. (1982) *Premature Babies*. Priam, New York.

New, W. (1985) Pulse oximetry. *Journal of Clinical Monitoring*, **1**(2), 126–9.

Norris, S., Campbell, L.A. & Brenkert, S. (1982) Nursing procedures and alterations in transcutaneous oxygen tension in premature infants. *Nursing Research*, **31**, 330–36.

Oehler, J.M. (1985) Examining the issue of tactile stimulation for preterm infants. *Neonatal Network*, **4**(3), 25–33.

Oehler, J.M., Eckerman, C.O. & Wilson, W.H. (1988) Social stimulation and the regulation of premature infants' state prior to term age. *Infant Behavior and Development*, **11**, 333–51.

Peters, K.L. (1992) Does routine nursing care complicate the physiologic status of the premature neonate with respiratory distress syndrome? *Journal of Developmental and Behavioral Pediatrics*, **8**, 68–76.

Powell, L.F. (1974) The effect of extra stimulation and maternal involvement on the development of low-birth-weight infants and on maternal behavior. *Child Development*, **45**, 106–13.

Rose, S.A., Schmidt, K. & Bridger, W. (1976) Cardiac and behavioral responsivity to tactile stimulation in premature and full-term infants. *Developmental Psychology*, **12**, 311–20.

Roy, S.C. (1984) *Introduction to Nursing: An Adaptation Model*, 2nd edn. Prentice-Hall, Englewood Cliffs, NJ.

Speidel, B.D. (1978) Adverse effects of routine procedures on preterm infants. *Lancet*, **i**, 864–6.

Tardy, T.J. & Volpe, J.J. (1982) Intraventricular hemorrhage in the premature infant. *Pediatric Clinics of North America*, **29**, 1077–104.

Weiss, S. (1979) The language of touch. *Nursing Research*, **28**, 76–80.

White-Traut, R. & Goldman, M.B.C. (1988) Premature infant massage: is it safe? *Pediatric Nursing*, **141**, 285–91.

# Chapter 3
# Long-term follow-up study of cerebral palsy children and coping behaviour of parents

TAIKO HIROSE, *RN, MS*
Doctoral student, School of Nursing, University of Washington, USA

and REIKO UEDA, *MA, DMS*
Professor of Human Development, University of Ibaraki, Ibaraki, Japan

The purpose of this study was to understand: (a) the feelings, thoughts and actions of parents at the time their children were diagnosed as having cerebral palsy; (b) the crisis periods in raising their children; (c) the important persons who supported the parents during the 'acceptance' phase; and (d) the roles of mothers and fathers in raising the children. The subjects were 28 mothers and 12 fathers who had sons or daughters with cerebral palsy. The latter offspring were aged 22–29 years at the time of this study. They were interviewed at their homes with a semi-structured method retrospectively. The results showed that most parents became aware of their children's disability in infancy and most of their children were diagnosed as having cerebral palsy by around two years of age. The mothers' reactions to the diagnosis were emotional and those of the fathers were realistic in coping with the problem. Although crisis periods arose throughout the periods of growth and development of the children, the infancy period was the more critical for mothers and the toddlerhood, school-age and adolescence periods were more critical for fathers. The important support people were the spouses. The mothers took care of the children while the fathers provided an income; however, some fathers withdrew from competing for achievement in their jobs.

## Introduction

Decades ago, researchers began documenting stress in families of handicapped children. More recently, investigators have observed how such families cope with their difficulties (Schilling *et al.*, 1985). Researchers on nursing began to study stress in families of handicapped children in the 1970s. Recently, they have investigated how such families cope with their children's problems. They have recognized the importance of social support for such families (MacElveen-Hoehn & Eyres, 1984; Brandt, 1984).

Recently, in Japan, the overall birth rate of babies with cerebral palsy has decreased from two out of 1000 to one out of 1000 births, due to an improvement in medical care, especially perinatal and neonatal medicine. However, the number of cerebral palsy babies with severe brain damage which involves severe mental retardation, epilepsy, and seizures has increased (Takahashi, 1992). Most of them are not in institutions, but they are enrolled in day care centres in all the prefectures in Japan. There are 73 day care centres for physically handicapped children, in addition to 72 institutions for them in Japan in 1990 (Health and Welfare Statistics Association, 1992).

### Team care

It is currently considered that comprehensive team approach in caring for them, facilitates the physical, psychological, emotional, and social develop-ment of cerebral palsy children. The team approach involves not only medical professionals, such as physicians, nurses, physiotherapists and occupational therapists, but also social workers, teachers, and caregivers, such as parents. Most team care is conducted in their homes in a community setting. In Japan, some children who used to live in institutions are now living at home and attending day care centres for training and treatment (Suganuma, 1992).

The role of nurses for handicapped children in Japan has been expanded from physical care in special hospitals or institutions to physical, mental and social care at home. The conditions of the care have changed from the time when nursing care for them was mainly offered in special hospitals or institutions for handicapped children in specific places in Japan. On the other hand, as Japanese family size has become smaller and nuclear families have increased, families with handicapped children need more support from health professionals such as nurses who provide physical, mental and social care at home, and organize social support for them. Additionally, a follow-up study on ADL (activities of daily living) in cerebral palsy children using the same subjects as in this study, was conducted in 1989 (Hirose & Gomi, 1992).

### *Purpose of the study*

The purpose of this study was to understand:

(1) The feelings, thoughts and actions of parents when their children are diagnosed as having cerebral palsy.

(2) The crisis periods in raising their children.
(3) The important persons who support the parents during the 'acceptance' phase.
(4) The roles of mothers and fathers in raising their children.

In this study, 'acceptance' is defined using Miller's (1968) definition as achieving mature understanding of their handicapped children. Miller categorized 'acceptance' into three stages. Stage 1 is disintegration and is that period of time when so much effort is being put into dealing with emotions that very little energy is left for coping effectively with the environment and carrying on. Stage 2 is adjustment, when parents suffer chronic sorrow, and partly accept and partly deny the retardation, all at the same time. Stage 3 is reintegration, when parents pull themselves back together and begin to function more effectively and more realistically.

## Subjects

The subjects were 28 mothers and 12 fathers with cerebral palsy sons and daughters (including one Lesh-Nyhan syndrome case). The ages of the offspring were from 22–29 years. Twelve of the mothers and the 12 fathers were couples.

The subjects of this study participated in an earlier study when 80 mothers and their cerebral palsy children (including one Lesh-Nyhan syndrome child) were admitted to the same national hospital and home for disabled children in Tokyo. During the earlier study, the children were toddlers or were of early school-age. However, only 28 mothers agreed to participate in this follow-up study in 1987. The study of the 12 fathers who agreed to participate in this study was conducted in 1988. The 28 offspring with cerebral palsy were born in Tokyo or in areas within commuting distance of Tokyo. At the time of this study, these adult children were living together with their families, except in one case where the father lived separately and three other cases where the fathers had died (the remaining 24 fathers were living together with their families).

## Method

The mothers and the fathers were interviewed by the same researcher. Both were interviewed with a semi-structured method retrospectively. The interviews took place in the homes of the families with some exceptions where the interviews took place in offices or coffee shops upon their request. The interview time of the mothers ranged from 1.33–3.5 hours (mean: 2.13

hours). The interview time of the fathers ranged from 1.0–1.5 hours (mean: 1.25 hours). The interview records of the mothers were written in running narrative form during and after the interviews. The records of the interviews of the fathers were recorded by a tape recorder.

## Questions

The content of the questions to the mothers was as follows:

(1) The present and previous social, mental and physical situations of mothers and their children with cerebral palsy.
(2) The mothers' process of acceptance of their children with cerebral palsy.
(3) The important persons who supported the mothers during difficulties, as well as details of the support.

The content of the questions to the fathers was as follows:

(1) The present and previous social, mental and physical situation of the fathers, especially the father's social situation during the child's growing-up period.
(2) The fathers' process of acceptance of the children with cerebral palsy.
(3) The important persons who supported the fathers during difficulties.
(4) The fathers' share in the raising of the child with cerebral palsy.

## *Results*

### Offspring with cerebral palsy

The current age of the offspring with cerebral palsy (CP) ranged from 22–29 years (mean: 24.9). There were 15 males and 13 females. Table 3.1 shows the types of cerebral palsy, birth order, sex, IQ (Tanaka-Binet Intelligence Test), LMA (lower motor age), UMA (upper motor age), ADL (activities of daily living) scores and life styles (Gomi, 1983; Hirose *et al.*, 1988). There were 14 athetoid types and 13 spastic types and one Lesh-Nyhan syndrome case. The IQ range was from 53–120 (mean: 91.5 ($n = 27$)) in toddlerhood, or in early school-age. Sixteen were the first born, 10 were the second, and the rest were the third. Ten of the families lived with grandparents (35.7%).

ADL was evaluated by a scoring method. ADL consisted of nine items in adolescence which included feeding, dressing, undressing, face washing, writing, bathing, walking, urinating and evacuating. For the cerebral palsy subjects in young adulthood, ADL included eight items: feeding, dressing, face washing, writing, bathing, walking, toileting and speech. The ADL scores ranged from 0–18 during adolescence, and those in young adulthood ranged from 0–16 since each item score ranged from 0–2 (Table 3.2).

**Table 3.1** Attributes of the offspring with CP.

| Name | Type of CP | Birth order | Sex | Age | LMA | UMA | IQ | Age | ADL score | Age | ADL score | Life style |
|------|-----------|-------------|-----|-----|-----|-----|-----|-----|-----------|-----|-----------|-----------|
| | | | | Toddlerhood–early school-age | | | | School-age–adolescence | | Young adulthood | | |
| K.I. | A | 1 | F | 5:4 | 2 | 4 | 120 | 15 | 2 | 24 | 1 | Day workshop |
| K.S. | S | 1 | F | 3:11 | 7 | 26 | 88 | 16 | 5 | 25 | 3 | Day workshop |
| S.Y. | A | 3 | F | 3:4 | 13 | 36 | 100 | 13 | 18 | 22 | 16 | Day workshop |
| S.O. | S | 2 | F | 4:2 | 11 | 39 | 90 | 16 | 16 | 25 | 10 | Day workshop |
| M.I. | S | 2 | F | 5:11 | 12 | 60 | 82 | 17 | 18 | 26 | 16 | Day workshop |
| S.Y. | A | 1 | F | 6:6 | 4 | 5 | 70 | 17 | 0 | 27 | 1 | Day workshop |
| H.H. | S | 1 | M | 5:7 | 9 | 60 | 110 | 18 | 17 | 27 | 15 | Day workshop |
| M.H. | A | 2 | M | 5:8 | 0 | 5 | 90 | 16 | 0 | 25 | 0 | Day workshop |
| M.O. | A | 1 | M | 4:1 | 9 | 4 | 100 | 16 | 0 | 25 | 6 | Day workshop |
| T.W. | S | 1 | M | 4:0 | 9 | 21 | 60 | 14 | 9 | 23 | 3 | Day workshop |
| T.M. | O | 2 | M | 3:2 | 2 | 7 | 53 | 14 | 0 | 22 | 1 | Day workshop |
| S.S. | S | 2 | M | 4:10 | 9 | 28 | 100 | 18 | 16 | 27 | 10 | Day workshop |
| H.S. | A | 1 | M | 4:1 | 13 | 18 | 89 | 15 | 10 | 24 | 9 | Day workshop |
| S.A. | S | 2 | F | 4:7 | 10 | 54.6 | 95 | 16 | 15 | 24 | 14 | Employed |
| A.O. | A | 1 | F | 4:10 | 15 | 33 | 110 | 19 | 18 | 28 | 16 | Employed |
| Y.O. | S | 1 | F | 4:1 | 12 | 24 | 100 | 15 | 17 | 24 | 15 | Employed |
| H.F. | A | 2 | M | 4:3 | 12 | 30 | 100 | 13 | 18 | 22 | 13 | Employed |
| H.Y. | S | 1 | M | 3:1 | 13 | 48 | 110 | 15 | 18 | 24 | 16 | Employed |
| M.H. | S | 1 | M | 4:0 | 16 | 42 | 99 | 14 | 17 | 22 | 15 | Employed |
| A.T. | A | 1 | M | 3:0 | 15 | 12 | 94 | 18 | 18 | 27 | 16 | Employed |
| F.S. | S | 3 | M | 3:6 | 11 | 45 | 100 | 14 | 17 | 22 | 15 | Employed |
| M.N. | A | 1 | F | 3:1 | 11 | 27 | 100 | 16 | 18 | 25 | 16 | Home |
| C.E. | A | 2 | F | 5:6 | 4 | 6 | 117 | 18 | 1 | 27 | 3 | Home |
| Y.S. | A | 1 | F | 4:9 | 12 | 24 | 100 | 16 | 18 | 25 | 14 | Home |
| J.K. | S | 1 | M | 3:2 | 15 | 25 | — | 16 | 18 | 25 | 16 | Home |
| Y.K. | A | 1 | M | 5:1 | 13 | 33 | 100 | 20 | 11 | 29 | 8 | Home |
| H.S. | S | 2 | F | 6:11 | 15 | 30 | 66 | 20 | 18 | 29 | 16 | Institutionalized |
| T.H. | A | 2 | M | 4:2 | 18.5 | 45 | 120 | 14 | 18 | 23 | 16 | Institutionalized |

A = Athetoid type; S = spastic type; O = other; LMA = lower motor age (month); UMA = upper motor age (month).

Table 3.3 shows life styles and ADL scores of the 28 adult children with cerebral palsy. Within the total group of offspring, there were eight (28.6%) who had occupations, including an office worker, computer programmer and a telephone operator. The remainder could not get jobs owing to their physical or mental handicaps, so were at home, worked in a day workshop or were institutionalized. Table 3.4 shows the ages, types of CP, birth orders, IQ, ADL scores in adulthood, and life styles for the 12 adult children with cerebral palsy of the 12 fathers who were interviewed in 1988. One son (8.3%) had a bachelor's degree and the rest graduated from high school for the physically handicapped. Four adult children with cerebral palsy (33.3%) had occupations.

**Table 3.2**   Definition of the scores.

| | |
|---|---|
| Independence | 2: capable by himself |
| | 1: needs partial help |
| | 0: needs help entirely |
| Writing | 2: able to write |
| | 1: not able to write in small letters |
| | 0: not able to write at all |
| Speech | 2: able to speak |
| | 1: able to speak with difficulty |
| | 0: not able to speak |
| Walking | 2: able to walk by himself |
| | 1: able to walk on crutches |
| | 0: moves by wheelchair |

**Table 3.3**   ADL and life styles of the adult children with CP ($n = 28$).

| Life style | ADL score | No. (%) |
|---|---|---|
| Employed | 13–16 | 8 (28.6) |
| Home | 3–6 | 5 (17.9) |
| Day workshop | 0–16 | 13 (46.4) |
| Institutionalized | 16 | 2 (7.1) |

**Table 3.4**   Attributes of the adult children with CP of the 12 fathers ($n = 12$).

| Name | Age in 1988 | Type of CP | Birth order | IQ in 3–6 years of age | ADL score in adulthood | Life style in 1988 |
|---|---|---|---|---|---|---|
| K.I. | 25 | A | 1 | 120 | 1 | Day workshop |
| K.S. | 26 | S | 1 | 88 | 3 | Day workshop |
| S.S. | 28 | S | 2 | 100 | 10 | Day workshop |
| T.H. | 24 | A | 2 | 120 | 16 | Day workshop |
| S.A. | 25 | S | 2 | 95 | 14 | Office worker |
| A.O. | 29 | A | 1 | 110 | 16 | Computer programmer |
| A.T. | 28 | A | 1 | 94 | 16 | Office worker |
| F.S. | 22 | S | 3 | 100 | 15 | Computer programmer |
| C.E. | 28 | A | 2 | 117 | 3 | Home |
| Y.S. | 26 | A | 1 | 100 | 14 | Home |
| Y.K. | 30 | A | 1 | 100 | 8 | Home |
| H.S. | 30 | S | 2 | 66 | 9 | Institutionalized |

### Mothers with cerebral palsy offspring

The ages of the 28 mothers ranged from 45–60 years old (mean: 52.8). Seventeen mothers were housewives and the rest had full-time jobs, part-time jobs, were in partnership with their husbands in a shop, or managed rental property. Four mothers whose sons or daughters had ADL scores ranging from 0–6 had lumbago due to caring for their sons or daughters. Table 3.5 shows the ages and levels of education of the 12 mothers whose husbands were interviewed in 1988. One mother (8.3%) had a bachelor's degree and 10 mothers (83.3%) had graduated from high school.

Table 3.6 shows when and how the mothers became aware of the developmental disabilities of their children with cerebral palsy. Table 3.7 shows when they were told of the cerebral palsy diagnosis. They became aware of the developmental disabilities of the children from the first month to the first year of age, and were told of the diagnosis by the child's third year of age. They had visited from two to eight facilities (mean: 4.1) including hospitals, public health centres and social welfare agencies to see and consult with doctors, and to have their child treated.

The mothers' reactions to the diagnosis were generally categorized as three types. The first was the pessimistic type. Mothers said such things as 'I couldn't think at the time', 'I wanted to commit suicide with the child' and 'I couldn't do anything but weep for a week'. The second was the optimistic type. They said such things as 'I suppose he will grow up with little or no handicap through treatment and rehabilitation'. The last category was the objective type. They said such things as 'I intended to raise the child the same as a normal child because there is no damage in intelligence' and 'I have thought about how to cope with the problem because I had suspected his disability'.

**Table 3.5**  Education of mothers of the 12 adult children (*n* = 12).

| Name | Age in 1987 | Education level |
|------|-------------|-----------------|
| K.I. | 52 | Bachelor's degree |
| K.S. | 45 | High school |
| S.S. | 60 | High school |
| T.H. | 55 | High school |
| S.A. | 52 | Junior high school |
| A.O. | 54 | High school |
| A.T. | 58 | High school |
| F.S. | 53 | High school |
| C.E. | 53 | High school |
| Y.S. | 47 | Junior high school |
| Y.K. | 58 | High school |
| H.S. | 56 | High school |

**Table 3.6**  Periods during which mothers become aware of their children's developmental disabilities and clues thereto (*n* = 28).

| Period (No.) (%) | Clues |
|---|---|
| 1–3 months of age (12) (42.9) | Slow visual following<br>Hyper-irritability to sound<br>Nuclear jaundice, convulsions<br>Hypertonic lower extremities<br>Dr noticed an abnormality of the infant<br>Dr noticed CP |
| 4–6 months of age (9) (32.1) | Head control (–)<br>Crying all day<br>Abnormality of lower extremities<br>Less development than twin brother |
| 7–12 months of age (7) (25.0) | Head control (–), sitting (–)<br>Floppy infant<br>Abnormality of lower extremities<br>Dr noticed an abnormality of the infant |

**Table 3.7**  When the mothers were told of the CP diagnosis (*n* = 27).

| Period (age) | No. (%) |
|---|---|
| 0–5 months | 4 (14.8) |
| 6–11 months | 6 (22.2) |
| 12–23 months | 13 (48.2) |
| 2–3 years | 4 (14.8) |

Twelve mothers (42.9%) were categorized as the pessimistic type. Thirteen mothers (46.4%) were categorized as the optimistic type and the remaining three mothers (10.7%) were categorized as the objective type. There was no relationship between the mothers' reaction and the ADL scores of the offspring at the time. For example, when the mother's reaction was pessimistic her offspring did not always have a low ADL score, and when the mother's reaction was optimistic her offspring did not always have a high ADL score.

Table 3.8 shows the most stressful period during the raising of the child. Twelve mothers (42.9%) had their most stressful period during the child's infancy due to the shock from the diagnosis, difficulties in the care of the child and the isolation. Seven mothers (25.0%) had their most difficult period during the child's toddlerhood, school-age and adolescence. Five mothers (17.9%) experienced their most stressful period after their child became 18 years of age. It seemed that the older the children were, the more difficult it was to cope with problems such as parental anxieties over what would

**Table 3.8**  When the mothers had the most stressful episodes (*n* = 28).

| Period | No. (%) |
|---|---|
| Infancy and early school-age (0–5 years) | 14 (50.0) |
| School-age and adolescence (6–17 years) | 5 (17.9) |
| After adolescence (18 years) | 5 (17.9) |
| NA | 4 (14.3) |

happen to the child after their death. Table 3.9 shows the persons who supported the mothers. Twenty-five mothers (89.3%) nominated their husbands as the important persons who supported them, and 16 mothers (57.1%) nominated mothers of children with the same handicap.

## The fathers of cerebral palsy offspring

The age of the 12 fathers ranged from 51–68 years (mean: 52.8). Table 3.10 shows the ages, levels of education and occupations of the fathers. Fifty per cent of the fathers had bachelor's degrees and eleven fathers (91.7%) graduated from high school. Two fathers whose daughters had low ADL scores ranging from 1–3 had lumbago due to caring for them.

There was a father who changed his job to enable him to take better care of his child with cerebral palsy. There were six fathers (50.0%) who adjusted their work to accommodate the care of the child, and four of the fathers abandoned promotion by refusing transfers in their companies, thus enabling better treatment of the child as well as better support for his family.

The fathers' reactions to the diagnosis of cerebral palsy were categorized into two types. The first category was the optimistic type. The second category was the objective and realistic type in coping with the problem. Two fathers (16.7%) were categorized as the optimistic type. Ten fathers (83.3%)

**Table 3.9**  Persons who supported the mothers (*n* = 28).

| Person | No. (%) |
|---|---|
| Husbands | 25 (89.3) |
| Mothers with a CP child | 16 (57.1) |
| Grandparents | 11 (39.3) |
| Relatives | 13 (46.4) |
| Doctors | 2 (7.1) |
| Children with CP | 1 (3.6) |
| Others | 5 (17.9) |

**Table 3.10**   Attributes of the fathers ($n = 12$).

| Name of offspring | Age of the father in 1988 | Education level | Occupation |
|---|---|---|---|
| K.I. | 53 | Bachelor's degree | Self-employed |
| K.S. | 51 | Junior high school | Self-employed |
| S.S. | 68 | Bachelor's degree | Retired (journalist) |
| T.H. | 58 | Junior college | White collar worker |
| S.A. | 59 | High school | Shop assistant |
| A.O. | 57 | High school | Cartoonist |
| A.T. | 63 | Bachelor's degree | Retired (teacher) |
| F.S. | 58 | High school | Self-employed |
| C.E. | 61 | Bachelor's degree | Self-employed (white collar worker) |
| Y.S. | 53 | Junior high school | Self-employed |
| Y.K. | 60 | Bachelor's degree | Management of his real estate (white collar worker) |
| H.S. | 63 | Bachelor's degree | Retired (railway worker) |

were categorized as objective and realistic. No one was categorized as pessimistic. Table 3.11 shows the periods when they had their most stressful experiences in raising the child. Eight fathers (66.7%) had their most stressful experience during the child's toddlerhood, school-age and adolescence. Nine fathers (75.0%) had a realistic understanding of the disabilities of the child in toddlerhood, school-age and adolescence.

Table 3.12 shows the important persons who have supported the 12 fathers and the 12 mothers. Nine fathers (75.0%) nominated their wives as the important persons who supported them. Two fathers (16.7%) indicated they relied on themselves: in contrast to the fathers, none of the mothers nominated themselves. The fathers did not nominate parents of similarly-handicapped children. All of the fathers participated in caring for their children. The fathers whose children had high ADL scores helped in keeping the child amused at home or went out with the child. The fathers whose children had lower ADL scores participated in helping with the child's toileting, bathing or feeding.

**Table 3.11**   When the fathers had the most stressful episodes ($n = 12$).

| Period | No. (%) |
|---|---|
| Infancy | 2 (16.7) |
| Toddlerhood, school-age and adolescence | 8 (66.7) |
| Currently | 1 (8.3) |
| Continuously | 1 (8.3) |

**Table 3.12** The important persons who supported the fathers and mothers ($n = 12$).

| Name of offspring | Persons who supported the fathers | Persons who supported the mothers |
|---|---|---|
| K.I. | Wife | Husband, mothers with a CP child |
| K.S. | Wife, union members, neighbours, father's sister | Husband |
| S.S. | Wife | Husband, grandparent |
| T.H. | Wife | Husband, mother's sister |
| S.A. | Himself | Husband, grandparent, mothers with a CP child |
| A.O. | Wife, father's brother-in-law | Husband, grandmother |
| A.T. | Wife | Husband, grandmother, mothers with a CP child |
| F.S. | Wife | Husband, mothers with a CP child |
| C.E. | Wife, volunteers | Husband, mothers with a CP child, volunteers |
| Y.S. | Child with CP, wife | Husband, relatives |
| Y.K. | Himself, child with CP, wife | Husband, grandfather, mother's friend |
| H.S. | Belief, wife | Husband, mother's friend, mother's brother, doctor |

## *Discussion*

### The feelings, thoughts and actions of parents with cerebral palsy children at the time of the diagnosis.

Accumulating evidence based upon human and animal studies suggests that there are biological differences in how males and females perceive and respond to social stimuli (Schilling *et al.*, 1985). Rossi (1984) argues that females have a predisposition for responding to 'an easier connection between feelings and their expression in words'. If wives and husbands perceive stressful events differently, then they will also use differing coping strategies to deal with perceived stress (Lazarus & Folkman, 1984). Stokes & Wilson (1984) suggested that females received more emotional support than males did.

In this study, there are different reactions at the time of the diagnosis for male and female parents with cerebral palsy offspring. The reactions of the mothers were categorized into three types: the pessimistic type, the optimistic type and the objective type. Most mothers were categorized as pessimistic and optimistic types. Therefore, most mothers seemed to be more emotional in their reactions.

In contrast to the mothers' emotional reactions, most fathers were categorized as objective and realistic. These differences in reactions between the mothers and the fathers may relate to different coping strategies in dealing with perceived stress.

## The crisis periods in raising their children

Researchers (Miller, 1968; Drotor *et al.*, 1975; Carreto 1981) suggested models which interpreted the processes of parents' acceptance of their disabled children over a short term. For example, Drotor and his colleagues suggested a hypothetical model for the course of parental reactions to the birth of a child with a congenital malformation during the period from seven days to 60 months after birth. They reported five stages, such as shock, denial, sadness and anger, adaptation, and re-organization. Keith (1973) suggested crisis periods occurred during the growth of the handicapped child. He described the four periods of crisis as:

(1) When parents first learn about or suspect the handicap.
(2) When, about age 5, a decision has to be reached as to whether the child will be able to go to ordinary school.
(3) When the handicapped person is ready to leave school.
(4) When the parents become older and are unable to care for their handicapped child.

It is important in nursing handicapped children and in supporting parents to know the process of acceptance and the crisis periods.

This study demonstrated that parents encountered various critical problems in addition to the crisis periods that Keith stated, even after the offspring had become adults. The important crisis periods for the mothers were during the child's infancy, while those for the fathers were during the child's toddlerhood, school-age and adolescence. It seemed that the mothers blamed themselves as the direct or indirect cause of the disability and experienced isolation. The mothers were supported by a few people, such as their husbands and relatives, during the infancy period of the child. When the mothers began to go to a special hospital, institution or school with the child they met many mothers experiencing similar problems and could get support from them. Additionally, the mothers seemed to have greater composure during the toddlerhood and early school-age stages when the child developed in motor activity. When the children came of age to leave school, the mothers experienced a lot of problems again.

In contrast to the mothers, the fathers had fewer difficulties during the infancy of the child. However, they had difficulties when their children reached toddlerhood, school-age and adolescence. The reason for the differences in difficult times between the mothers and the fathers might be explained by the different roles in the child-rearing behaviour of the parents.

## The important persons who supported the parents

Faber (1959) noticed marital integration in a family with a severely mentally regarded child, and Friedrich (1979) suggested that marital satisfaction was the best predictor of the coping behaviour of mothers with handicapped children. Mardiros (1982) and Haggerty (1980) suggested that a parent support group made up mostly of mothers with disabled children was the most helpful.

In this study, the most helpful persons for the mothers and fathers were their spouses. Other mothers facing similar problems were the next most important sources of support for the mothers. Additionally, both the mothers and the fathers were supported by their relatives. The mothers had a larger number of supporters than the fathers. The difference between the mothers and the fathers seems to be that women under stress seek comfort and advice from others because of a personal sense of how much help they could receive from others, and because they developed affectionately richer friendships than the men. The men tended to use coping strategies which were consonant with their social role. Thus, the fathers tended to keep their problems to themselves (Byrne & Cunningham, 1985). This study indicates the importance of the marital relationship as support for the coping behaviour of the parents when experiencing difficulties, because 11 couples (91.7%) nominated their spouses as the persons who supported them. There was one exception in which a mother nominated her husband but the father nominated himself.

## The role of the mothers and fathers in raising the children

Several researchers (Cooke & Lawton, 1984; Byrne & Cunningham, 1985; Schilling *et al.*, 1985) indicated that the major burden was carried by mothers in a family with a handicapped child. Again, in this study, the major burden of raising the child with cerebral palsy was carried by the mothers.

Mothers with little support provided the extraordinary care required by a cerebral palsy infant, and therefore they had their most stressful period during the child's infancy. One mother said, 'I sang a nursery song for my baby by myself in my house every day because I didn't have friends to whom I could tell my difficulties, and my only pleasure was a drive with my husband and baby on Sunday'. After the children entered school for the physically handicapped, most mothers were going to the school with the children every day. One of the mothers said that she carried the child on her back to the school.

The mothers' role seemed to be crucial in caring for the child and the family. The father's role seemed to be supporting the mothers and the family. Four of the 12 fathers abandoned promotion in their companies when they refused to be transferred so that their children could be treated by the best doctors using high-level medical care in Tokyo. This was an alternative to competing for achievement in their jobs. One of the four fathers said, 'Fathers with non-handicapped children can keep a balance with their family and work easily, but fathers with handicapped children like me do it with many difficulties and afflictions'. What he said reveals the difficult role of the fathers with handicapped children.

Many papers and articles have been published on the role of the father in child development (Lamb, 1976; Hanson 1985–6), but research papers on the role of the fathers with handicapped children are few, especially in Japan. Further research is needed.

The parents in this study seemed to be coping very well under the circumstances. They had good health and intelligence for raising their children with cerebral palsy. They had intimate marital relationships, with a few exceptions. Supportive human resources and social resources were available because they lived in Tokyo or in the suburbs of Tokyo. They had flexible coping behaviours for raising children with cerebral palsy because the parents were not socially isolated. Functions, such as good health, intelligence, rich human and social resources, and flexible coping behaviour identified in this study, also seemed important in their agreement to continue participating in this study.

## Conclusion

Studies from direct observational methods and longitudinal studies are needed to develop better nursing care for the families with handicapped children. Yet, this study on handicapped children and the family offers a longitudinal perspective over a long span of nursing care from the child's infancy to young adulthood.

## Acknowledgement

The authors would like to express sincere gratitude and appreciation to Dr Shigeharu Gomi for his co-operation.

## References

Brandt, P.A. (1984) Social support and negative life events of mothers with developmentally delayed children. *Birth Defects*, **20**(5), 205–44.

Byrne, E.A. & Cunningham, C.C. (1985) The effects of mentally handicapped children on families – a conceptual review. *Journal of Child Psychology and Psychiatry*, **26**(6), 847–64.

Carreto, V. (1981) Maternal responses to an infant with cleft lip and palate. A review of literature. *MCN*, **10**(3), 197–206.

Cooke, K. & Lawton, D. (1984) Informal support for the carers of disabled children. *Child: care, health and development*, **10**(2), 67–79.

Drotor, D., Baskiewicz, A., Irvin, N., Kennell, J. & Klaus, M. (1975) The adaptation of parents to the birth of an infant with a congenital malformation: a hypothetical model. *Pediatrics*, **56**(5), 710–17.

Faber, B. (1959) Effects of severely mentally retarded children on family integration. *Monographs of the Society for Research in Child Development*, **24**(2).

Friedrich, W.N. (1979). Predictors of the coping behavior of mothers of handicapped children. *Journal of Consulting and Clinical Psychology*, **47**(6), 1140–41.

Gomi, S. (1983) A follow-up study on cerebral palsy. In *Cerebral Palsy* (ed. N. Tsuyama), pp. 356–80. Kyoudoisho, Tokyo.

Gomi, S. (1992). Longitudinal prognosis of cerebral palsy. In *Cerebral Palsy: Pediatric Rehabilitation*, vol. 1 (eds H. Iwakura, C. Iwatani & N. Doi), pp. 47–76. Ishiyaku, Tokyo.

Haggerty, R.J. (1980) Life stress, illness, and social support. *Developmental Medicine and Child Neurology*, **22**, 391–400.

Hanson, S.M. (1985–6) Father–child relationship. *Marriage & Family Review*, **9**(3–4), 135–50.

Health and Welfare Statistics Association (1992). Physical and mental disability. *Journal of Health and Welfare Statistics*, **39**(9), 171.

Hirose, T., Gomi, S. & Ueda, R. (1988) ADL in cerebral palsied children: a long-term follow-up study. *Bulletin of Tokyo Metropolitan College of Allied Medical Sciences*, **1**, 41–7.

Hirose, T. & Gomi, S. (1992). A long-term follow-up study on ADL in cerebral palsied children. *Bulletin of Tokyo Metropolitan College of Allied Medical Sciences*, **5**, 65–74.

Keith, R.M. (1973) The feelings and behavior of parents of handicapped children. *Developmental Medicine and Child Neurology*, **15**, 524–7.

Lamb, M.E. (1976) *The Role of the Father in Child Development*, pp. 1–6. John Wiley, New York.

Lazarus, R.S. & Folkman, S. (1984) *Stress, Appraisal, and Coping*. Springer, New York.

MacElveen-Hoehn, P. & Eyres, J.S. (1984) State of the art in relation to families and children. *Birth Defects*, **20**(5), 11–43.

Mardiros, M. (1982) Mothers of disabled children: a study of parental stress. *Nursing Papers*, **14**(3), 47–56.

Miller, L.G. (1968) Toward a greater understanding of the parents of mentally retarded children. *Journal of Pediatrics*, **73**(5), 699–705.

Rossi, A.S. (1984) Gender and parenthood. *American Sociological Revue*, **49**, 1–9.

Schilling, R.F., Schilling, R.F. II., Schinke, S.P. & Kirkham, M.A. (1985) Coping with a handicapped child: differences between mothers and fathers. *Social Science and Medicine*, **21**(8), 857–63.

Stokes, J.P. & Wilson, D.G. (1984) The inventory of socially supportive behaviors: dimensionary, prediction, and gender differences. *American Journal of Community Psychology*, **12**(1), 53–69.

Suganuma, I. (1992). Care management for severe physically and mentally handicapped children. In *Cerebral Palsy: Pediatric Rehabilitation*, vol. 1 (eds H. Iwakura, C. Iwatani, & N. Doi) pp. 195–215. Ishiyaku, Tokyo.

Takahashi, T. (1992). Development of the medical care for cerebral palsy children, and changes in the definition and diagnosis of cerebral palsy. In *Cerebral Palsy: Pediatric Rehabilitation*, vol. 1 (eds H. Iwakura, C. Iwatani, & N. Doi), pp. 1–18. Ishiyaku, Tokyo.

# Chapter 4
# Changing attitudes towards families of hospitalized children from 1935 to 1975: a case study

JUDITH YOUNG, *RN, MScN*

Tutor, Faculty of Nursing, University of Toronto, 50 St George Street, Toronto, Ontario M5S 1A1, Canada

The introduction of 'open' visiting and family involvement in the care of hospitalized children created a revolution in the care of children in hospitals. This historical study utilized the situation at the Hospital for Sick Children, Toronto (HSC), as a case study illustrating change. Although psychological research provided a strong rationale for including families in the care of hospitalized children, change occurred slowly. In this regard, HSC was typical of many children's hospitals. However, there seemed to be a significant failure to learn from innovations elsewhere. Paediatric nurses, in particular, were slow to encourage family visiting and participation in care.

## Introduction

The inclusion of families on the wards of paediatric hospitals was a radical change occurring only in recent decades. Why were most children's hospitals so slow to welcome families? A historical perspective on this question offers information and insight which may help to guide future practice. The situation at the Hospital for Sick Children, Toronto (HSC), Canada's oldest and largest paediatric hospital, provides a case study which illustrates the changing pattern of family visiting and participation in the care of children.

HSC has been known since the late nineteenth century for its innovative medical and surgical treatment. However, the hospital was reluctant to adopt innovations in psychosocial aspects of care and, in particular, was slow to allow families greater access to their children (Young, 1987). Certain paediatric hospitals did pioneer acceptance of families in their wards during the 1950s, although most hospitals caring for sick children did not welcome families until much later.

For many years, HSC professionals appeared to lack conviction that change was necessary. This chapter attempts to explain why a leading paediatric institution progressed so slowly towards creating a more humane environment for its patients and, in particular, assesses the role of HSC nurses in promoting or retarding change.

## Scope of the study

Primary sources of information for this historical study included HSC Annual Reports, internal newsletters, memorandums, regulations and minutes of the Medical Advisory Board. Nurses, doctors and former patients and parents provided sources of oral history. Further perspectives on nursing attitudes and beliefs were gained by reviewing issues of the *Canadian Nurse* which were published during the period studied. Research papers and books on the psychosocial welfare of children in hospital yielded secondary source material.

The years 1935 to 1975 were studied because major change towards inclusion of families occurred at HSC and elsewhere within this period. For example, in 1935 public ward visiting at HSC was restricted to one hour on Sunday afternoons – a practice which had been in existence for decades. Regulations were considerably less restrictive for the small number of private patients (HSC, 1928). Such regulations were the norm for children's hospitals at the time. On visiting days, parents sat by their child's bed. Infants were viewed through a window. Visitors also had minimal interaction with nursing or medical staff. But, by 1975 most wards at HSC allowed unrestricted visiting by parents who participated increasingly in the actual care of their children.

Although a major focus of the study was on the role of nursing in promoting or retarding change, a brief assessment of the effects of medical influences was also necessary. In addition, information concerning the social milieu of the hospital and trends in child psychology and child-rearing practices provided background data significant to the course of events.

## *Class differences shape attitudes towards families*

Hospitals for children, an innovation in the nineteenth century, were founded for the sick poor. Children received care and nourishment, but moral training and guidance were of equal importance (Vogel, 1980). HSC was no exception. It was founded in 1875 by a group of upper-middle-class women for 'sick, destitute and friendless children ... [and] sick children whose parents owing to poverty are unable to attend them' (HSC, 1876).

A wide social gulf separated the early lady managers and the families they served. Though great compassion was shown for the plight of poor families, hospital personnel were considered superior caregivers and parents were limited to twice weekly visits (Young, 1990). Those initially recruited to provide nursing care at HSC were untrained, respectable working-class women; however, with the creation of a training school in 1886, nurses came increasingly from the middle classes. Thus, the social gulf between patients and caregivers was perpetuated at HSC for many decades.

As the hospital expanded, control of infection became a major issue and provided a scientific rationale for further visiting restrictions. With the admission of infants after 1900, fear of cross-infection led to the creation, in 1914, of cubicled infant wards based on a Paris model. Parents were allowed to view their babies, but not to enter the cubicles.

HSC annual reports document that the majority of patients were in the public ward category until the expansion of hospital insurance schemes in the 1950s. Private patients were accommodated from 1892, but constituted a very small minority. They were, however, granted a particular privilege, that of daily visiting. Similar distinctions in visiting were routine in other hospitals and were not questioned at the time (Rosenberg, 1987).

Information from the 1930s illustrates aspects of public and private care which highlight the class distinctions of this era. W. Hawke, MD, a paediatric resident at HSC in 1935, graphically described his perception of care on the public wards. In the admitting department the child was separated from the parent, examined, and sent to the ward. Hawke likened the system to that of a Chinese laundry where packages were left and then picked up by the parent when treatment was complete. On visiting day, parents lined up to see the intern on duty; they would, of course, rarely see a staff doctor. 'Most striking' was visitation on the infant and isolation wards where parents viewed children from outside balconies regardless of the 'inclement weather' (Hawke, personal communication, February 1987).

### Enlarged facilities for private patients

Enlarged facilities for private patients were opened in 1935. This move was in keeping with the trend towards encouraging the patronage of middle-class patients and, thus, greater respectability for the hospital. The new HSC private wing was described as 'a fairyland of a hospital', with pink and white checked gingham curtains, easy chairs and hooked rugs creating a 'homelike atmosphere' (New private wing, 1935). A nursery for infants was included. This facility contrasted sharply with the stark public wards. A photograph from the late 1930s depicted a ward with no drapes, chairs or even toys (Braithwaite, 1974).

Regulations from the 1940s list private ward visiting as daily from 2.30

p.m. to 8 p.m. (HSC, 1948). A 1938 memorandum gives information on charges for overnight stay of parents on the private units (Bower, 1938). The different regulations seem to indicate that parents of private patients were not considered an infection hazard. Dr Hawke noted that, in this era, parents were considered a 'necessary nuisance', so probably a small group, similar in social class to the staff, was easier to tolerate (Hawke, personal communication, February 1987).

In 1951 a new Hospital for Sick Children was completed, but the new building was structured like the old one as far as the care of young children was concerned. The fourth floor (for infants and children up to two years) consisted of cubicles with glassed-in viewing corridors, 'so that parents may see but not come in contact with the patient at any time' (Bower 1951. The press emphasized equality of care of public and private patients in the new facility, though this certainly did not include equal access of parents to the hospital or to information from doctors. Equal visiting rights did not come until the 1960s. By then a government plan provided most Ontario families with hospital insurance, and research in child psychology had slowly affected practices in children's hospitals, including HSC (Young, 1992).

## Influence of child psychology

The idea of allowing mothers to stay with their hospitalized children was advocated in the 1920s by James Spence, a British paediatric surgeon. Spence (1951) considered this approach to be a 'humane, happy and satisfactory method of nursing sick children, particularly those under four years old'. His method, however, was not generally publicized until research gave it credibility.

Psychological research, starting in the 1940s, provided powerful evidence of the effects of 'hospitalism', a term used by American researcher Spitz (1945), and 'maternal deprivation' described by British psychologist Bowlby (1953) in his report to the World Health Organization. Children in orphanages were the initial focus of research, but it was hypothesized that children in hospitals were likewise at risk.

Robertson (1953), an associate of Bowlby, filmed the stay of a 2-year-old in hospital, and identified the stages of what he termed 'separation anxiety'. In the United States, Prugh *et al.* (1953) conducted an influential study of two groups of hospitalized children. This research demonstrated the beneficial effects of daily visiting and a play programme on the mental health of young children. Reformers promoted the idea of close involvement of the mother in the child's hospital care and the use of play as a therapeutic tool. But these ideas were slow to be adopted at HSC and elsewhere.

**Delayed influence**

The delayed influence of research can be explained in part by the prevailing beliefs regarding child care at that time. Historian Strong-Boag (1976) described the pervasive influence of professional advice to parents. In Toronto, HSC physician-in-chief Alan Brown published a popular manual for parents entitled *The Normal Child*. This book went through many editors between 1923 and 1958 with minimal revision of ideas. Brown stressed the importance of rigid feeding and sleeping schedules for infants. Strict schedules were the outcome of the scientific feeding movement which had gained ascendancy in the 1920s (Spock, 1946).

Brown (1932) also instructed parents to handle their infants as little as possible, so that they would learn to amuse themselves. He stated that the infant's nervous system was delicate and advised against lively play and undue stimulation. Kissing the infant was 'purely indulgence for the adult' and considered an infection hazard (Brown 1932).

Professionals in the 1930s thought independence from mother was critical even in the very young. A psychiatrist, writing in the *Canadian Nurse*, advised readers that mothers frequently hinder their children from gaining 'emotional independence' (Gee 1938). A period in hospital, away from mother, would therefore not be considered harmful. Child care practices which emphasized rigid schedules and strict discipline supported existing styles of ward management. Nursing rounds were 'like a military review of the troops' with children tucked neatly in bed (Rolstin, 1972).

By the early 1950s, however, new ideas in child psychology were beginning to affect child care in North American and British homes. Rigid feeding, sleep and toileting schedules were relaxed, and far less emphasis was placed on eradicating such habits as thumb sucking. American paediatrician Benjamin Spock (1957) thought that the change in philosophy with regard to spoiling amounted to 'a revolution'. Parents were now encouraged to hold their babies in order to provide comfort and loving attention, a practice previously thought inadvisable except at feeding time.

Alan Brown's influence may have helped to delay the spread of such new ideas in Toronto. He remained dedicated to strict feeding schedules and the pre-eminence of medical advice in child rearing (Brown & Robertson, 1958). A Toronto newspaper noted that a special project of the HSC Women's Auxiliary was the making of restraint jackets 'to keep baby thumbs from rosebud mouths'. The jackets were much in demand outside the hospital, as HSC doctors recommended them to parents (Women's groups, 1952).

Psychological research relating to hospitalization proliferated, however, and in 1965 Vernon *et al.* reviewed over 200 papers and books on the subject. Some of the most influential work in this area was carried out by British psychologist, Robertson. His films and writings became the most well-known in Canada. Robertson based a memorandum to the British Ministry of Health, for the Platt Committee, on his study of hospitalized children. In 1959 this committee produced the frequently cited Platt Report in which a recommendation was made that mothers of very young children requiring hospitalization be admitted with them. Open visiting, recreation programmes and psychosocial training of nurses and physicians were also recommended (Ministry of Health, 1959).

## HSC nurses promote and resist change

There is strong evidence that nurses at HSC both promoted and resisted changes which would allow parents greater access to their children and participation in their care. Resistance to change was also widespread among paediatric nurses elsewhere. Robertson (1970) was particularly scathing in his comments on the British Paediatric Nurses' Association, and their poor response to suggestions from the Platt Committee. Lamb & Solomon (1965) noted that acceptance of families required a major restructuring of the social system of the wards, and also required nurses to share the satisfaction derived from caring for a sick child. Dimock (1959), a Canadian psychologist, thought that many paediatric nurses satisfied their own emotional needs through the dependence and affection of their patients.

The climate in hospitals was not good for introducing new ideas supporting a radical change in the care of children. Nurses were trained to obey orders, carry out procedures and not to question or make judgement decisions. Many nurses truly felt they were better able to provide care than parents. It was also widely thought that children adjusted best to hospital without family visiting. The fact that most children became quiet and resigned when parents were not present was taken to be proof of this conclusion. It was only in later years that withdrawn behaviour was seen as a form of regression due to confinement and separation from family. In the 1940s the child who became agitated and visibly distressed was considered poorly adjusted due to lack of home discipline (Filer, 1943).

### Nursing educators

Nursing educators at HSC attempted to include new content related to child care into the curriculum. R. McCamus, a 1959 Children's Hospital graduate, was introduced to Bowlby's theory of maternal deprivation in classes given by a teacher from the Institute of Child Study in Toronto. Later, as a nursing instructor at HSC in the early 1960s, she showed students Robertson's film *A Two Year Old Goes to Hospital* and discussed separation anxiety. But, at the same time, she stated that hospital regulations severely restricted visiting on the wards, a policy in opposition to the ideas she taught (McCamus, personal communication, February 1987).

However, some nurses at HSC were sensitized to the need for change by incidents they experienced in their work. L. Ashton, a 1935 graduate, recalled her student experience on the isolation unit. A small boy with poliomyelitis became more agitated whenever he was left alone. She felt some of the subsequent deterioration in his condition could have been avoided if he had had the support of his parents. Later, in the 1950s, as a surgical head nurse, she tried to influence colleagues to recommend increased parental visiting (Ashton, personal communication, January 1987).

In the early 1950s a few nurses on the infant wards at HSC wanted less restrictions on visiting with parents allowed into infant cubicles. But E. Atkins, a head nurse who recalled the situation in 1951, said that requests for such a change, submitted through the nursing office, made no headway. She felt requests were not supported by nursing supervisory staff at this time. Also, nurses were not in agreement with the idea of expanded visiting; for example, some disregarded hospital policies and let mothers into infant cubicles, while others did not and were annoyed at such infractions of the rules (Atkins, personal communication, February 1987). Dr Hawke described an 'underground movement' where some nurses were prepared to take matters into their own hands (Hawke, personal communication, February 1987).

### Struggle for daily visiting

The nurses who wished to expand visiting at HSC were supported by a few junior physician colleagues (B. Greenleaf, personal communication, March 1987). There is, however, overwhelming evidence that throughout the 1950s senior medical staff remained actively opposed to such change. The HSC situation can be contrasted with that at Montreal Children's Hospital where extension of visiting and innovations in psychosocial care occurred throughout the decade (Dimock, 1959; James 1956). HSC practice was certainly typical of most institutions at the time, but the failure to recognize innovations elsewhere seems atypical for a leading paediatric institution.

Newspaper articles present the views of medical staff in the 1950s. In the *Toronto Star Weekly* an HSC doctor is quoted as saying that 'rarely does hospitalization create emotional problems in well-adjusted children from stable homes' (Your child in hospital, 1952). *Maclean's Magazine* noted the difference of opinion between doctors at HSC and the Montreal Children's Hospital. Montreal was about to provide overnight accommodation for some mothers, while HSC continued severe restrictions on parental visiting (How to help, 1956).

The minutes of the HSC Medical Advisory Board indicate that requests to increase visiting privileges were turned down throughout the 1950s (HSC, 1953, 1957). According to these minutes, the decision in 1957 to refuse daily visiting appeared to be greatly influenced by the chief of surgery. Requests for change were supported by some nurses, psychiatrist W. Hawke and the hospital superintendent (B. Greenleaf, personal communication, March 1987). However, official visiting policy remained unchanged for a further few years.

## Daily visiting introduced

In 1961 daily visiting on the public wards was finally introduced at HSC, though confined to three hours in the afternoons. All-day visiting, 11 a.m. to 8 p.m., was introduced in 1965. It is difficult to find out by what process daily visiting was actually achieved; but in 1961 the new superintendent (director), John Law, sent a questionnaire to parents asking for their reactions to their child's hospital experience. A summary of the responses was given to the Medical Advisory Committee (HSC, 1961). It seems likely that Law, by use of the questionnaire, hoped to gather data supporting changes in visiting policy.

Head nurse, V. Broe, recalled a directive from Law announcing daily afternoon visiting. This appeared to be an administrative decision which medical staff were expected to accept (Broe, personal communication, February 1987). Starr (1982) noted that, with increased complexity of internal organization, authority in American hospitals passed from physicians to administrators. At HSC the power of the Medical Advisory Board was greatly reduced in 1958 when it was changed to committee status with a function to provide broad advice (HSC, 1958).

The isolation wards at HSC were governed by regulations distinct from those of the rest of the hospital and, prior to 1965, no visiting was allowed unless a child was critically ill. The need to control the spread of infection was a historical fact underlying restrictions on visiting imposed decades earlier throughout children's hospitals. Infection control became a major issue as hospitals expanded and also provided a scientific rationale, in addition to other reasons discussed, for the visiting restrictions.

Many doctors and nurses still felt special regulations should remain in isolation wards despite the advent of antibiotics and immunization which made stringent control of visiting no longer necessary. The head of the infectious service at HSC, trained in a different era, could not adapt his thinking to such a major change as allowing parents into the isolation wards. When he did permit parents to visit in 1965, it was a direct result of strong nursing pressure. In particular, this came from H. Palmer, nursing supervisor of the medical wards (Palmer, personal communication, January 1987).

*Families receive a mixed welcome*

By the late 1960s many paediatric institutions had introduced all-day visiting, while some centres, notably in Britain, allowed mothers to 'live in'. But the British experience emphasized that legislation did not alter attitudes and that change was fraught with many difficulties. For instance, Meadows (1969), described the plight of the 'captive mother', who was allowed to live-in but was 'on trial', not particularly welcomed and afraid to negotiate time away from her child's bedside. Although given scant information, she was afraid to ask questions and routine procedures provoked anxiety. Meadows, a psychiatrist, considered that only nursing and medical acceptance of parents on the wards, and the nurse's willingness to share the care of the child, could alleviate this situation.

It was important for nurses to learn new skills in the area of human relations. There was much resentment directed towards anxious parents simply because nurses did not know how to talk to them (Lamb & Solomon, 1965). Parents were expected to hide their anxiety, a totally unrealistic expectation. Most nurses in the 1960s and early 1970s were still the products of a rigid procedure-orientated training system, and some were not willing to change their practice.

Successful change required the paediatric nurse to advance in other ways. Knowledge of physical growth and development had been taught for some time; but in order to help the child and family cope with illness, an understanding of more abstract theories regarding stages of emotional and intellectual growth was necessary. This was difficult for nurses unless their minds were open to learning and change.

On the HSC wards of the late 1960s and early 1970s, attitudes and practices towards families varied. There were no written standards of nursing care until the mid-1970s. Prior to this, a ward's philosophy regarding open visiting, overnight stay of parents and parental involvement in care depended on the individual head nurse, the influence of her supervisor, and the presence or absence of a supporting team from other disciplines. Although the three nursing supervisors of the medical, surgical and infant wards appeared to hold similar beliefs regarding family involvement in care, they did not work together to promote a hospital-wide approach. This lack of cohesiveness led to widely divergent practices.

### Initiating change

A variety of factors helped nurses initiate change on the medical wards at HSC. These included the involvement of social work and psychiatry in patient and family care and an influential nursing supervisor who, in the early 1970s, introduced specialist nurses in mental health and haematology.

The unit caring for children with leukaemia was the first to encourage overnight stay by providing roll-away cots for parents (Cragg, 1969). The development in the early 1970s of a strong psychosocial team approach for dialysis/transplant patients illustrates progress, in this speciality, towards family-focused care. Leadership, in this instance, was provided by a psychiatrist and social worker. However, physician support was a crucial factor and nurses were eager to develop their skills in working with families.

Although some surgical nurses at HSC were anxious for change, for many years there was both a lack of support and active opposition from surgeons to increased parental visiting. This was particularly true of the Tonsil Suite where parents were excluded from visiting right up to the early 1970s.

In the mid-1960s nurses became increasingly concerned about a group of long-term patients: those with chronic tracheostomies. These children lived in the hospital for months, even years, and the effects of maternal deprivation and lack of environmental stimulation were evident (Mitchell, 1968). Nurses formed links with psychiatry and social work despite opposition from ENT surgeons who resented interference in the care of the children (J.J. VanLeeuwen, personal communication, January 1987). Nurses became part of a 'self-appointed' interdisciplinary committee, which initiated improvements in the care of long-term patients. This committee eventually achieved official status as the Child Care Practices Committee (A. Evans, personal communication, January 1987).

A study was conducted on the surgical wards at HSC in 1968. The investigator, a head nurse, asked parents how they wished to participate, and asked nurses what they felt parents were capable of doing. Most parents wished to do more than nurses would allow (MacDonald, 1969). The study became the basis of a long-term project, the Family Centred Care Project, which sought to change nursing attitudes towards parent participation. The project was implemented on the surgical wards over the next five years by A. Evans, a young nurse who had recently returned to HSC after furthering her education. She recalled that the more familiar she became with the literature on the effects of separation, the more she felt compelled to change the situation at HSC.

Progress was slow. Head nurses varied in their reception to new ideas, and Evans noted that those who were rigid and controlling erected many barriers. Some were polite to her, but then proceeded to sabotage certain measures designed to give parents greater access to unit facilities. Some nurses resented the disruption of routines and the interference with their mothering role. But as staff became accustomed to the presence of families in the wards, most accepted this change. The project co-ordinator expanded her role to include orientation of new staff to family participation in care and the education of other hospital workers (Evans, personal communication, January 1987).

Introduction of family participation on the infant wards proceeded very slowly, even though the supervisor of these wards and a few head nurses supported parental involvement. Perhaps the long-held HSC practice of segregation of infants in cubicles with viewing corridors was too ingrained. Space was limited, and some nurses considered this to be a valid reason to control the expansion of visiting.

Although parents were allowed increased daily visiting in 1965, and could go inside cubicles to hold their infants, overnight visitation was not permitted. By the early 1970s the neonatal unit, which cared for premature and critically ill newborns, was allowing parents to visit at any time. M. McLean, the head nurse of this unit from 1971, later said that in her mind parents were not visitors and should have free access to their infants.

However, some nursing staff had difficulty sharing their nurturing role with parents. Certain nurses had great emotional investment in some infants and would attempt to defer transfer of the baby to another ward or to a hospital nearer home (McLean, personal communication, April 1987).

Although nurses at HSC did assist parents to become increasingly involved in the care of their children between 1970 and 1975, there was no universal commitment to this practice on the wards. The three most senior nursing supervisors supported the inclusion of families but were perhaps deterred by the size of the institution and did not work together to promote a co-ordinated nursing philosophy and plan.

Resistance to change among nurses at HSC remained strong. Generally, those who were more enlightened needed the support of other disciplines such as social work and psychiatry. When this was forthcoming, nurses promoted practice which encouraged the increasing participation of families.

## Conclusions

The inclusion of families on the wards of children's hospitals marked a major advance in the humane care of hospitalized children. The Hospital for Sick Children, Toronto, provided a case study illustrating this changing pattern of care. The acceptance of families at HSC was slow, though typical of many hospitals where children were admitted. However, it is surprising that HSC, as a major paediatric institution, failed to follow the leadership of those hospitals that pioneered family participation.

There appear to be a variety of reasons why Canada's oldest and largest paediatric hospital was so slow to welcome families. At HSC, where medical science was paramount, major psychological research on the institutionalization of children appeared to have little impact on medical staff. In fact, there was continued active opposition from physicians and surgeons to the liberalization of family visiting. Nurses were introduced to the work of Bowlby and Robertson during their training, but teachers had little influence on the wards. There, nursing opinion was strongly divided, a factor which reduced the power of nurses to influence change.

Eventually, the power to set visiting policies passed from physicians to HSC administration, and medical and nursing staff bowed to change. It is the author's opinion that the need to improve public relations, rather than the impact of psychological research, led most HSC physicians to accept family presence on the wards. Nurses, however, did increasingly accept the ideas of psychological research as a rationale for change.

## Effect on policies

Research on the effects of institutionalization did finally affect policies at HSC. The humanitarian nature of the reforms, and the logic of the idea that sick children needed their families, helped to make the acceptance of ideas from psychological research inevitable. The delayed impact of this research illustrates the fact that intellectual ideas are often slowly assimilated, even though they are humanitarian and the product of logical reasoning. Many cling to old ideas because they refuse to believe the evidence of research or are unable to face the insecurity that accompanies change.

There is strong evidence that nurses at HSC both promoted and resisted change in attitudes towards families. Resistance to family presence was widespread among nurses elsewhere, too. Change required a major restructuring of the social system of hospital wards. This was difficult for many nurses to accept, and impossible for some.

Although more progress was necessary to advance the integration of families into the care of children at HSC, by 1975 significant change was underway. The early movement for change had been reluctant and fragmented. But by 1975 the indications were that families at HSC were about to become an integral part of the institution.

## *Acknowledgement*

The research on which this chapter is based was partially supported by a grant from the Hospital for Sick Children, Toronto, Nursing Alumnae.

## *References*

Bower, J. (1938, June 28). Unpublished memo. Accounting File, HSC Archives, Toronto
Bower, J. (1951) Serving sick children. *The Canadian Hospital*, **28**(2), 36–43.
Bowlby, J. (1953) *Child Care and the Growth of Love*, pp. 13–20. Penguin, Harmondsworth, Middlesex.

Braithwaite, M. (1974) *Sick Kids: The Story of the Hospital for Sick Children*, photo, 'A ward in the fifth hospital', following p. 161. McClelland & Stewart, Toronto.

Brown, A. (1932) *The Normal Child*, 3rd edn, p. 223. McClelland & Stewart, Toronto.

Brown, A. & Robertson, B. (1958) *The Normal Child*, 5th edn., pp. 14, 37. Harlequin, Toronto.

Cragg, C. (1969) The child with leukaemia. *Canadian Nurse*, **65**(10), 30– 34.

Dimock, H.G. (1959) *The Child in Hospital: a Study of His Emotional and Social Wellbeing*, pp. 33–57. MacMillan, Toronto.

Filer, M.M. (1943) Nursing aspects of chorea. *Canadian Nurse*, **39**, 813–25.

Gee, M.M. (1938) Personality development of the pre-school child. *Canadian Nurse*, **34**, 706–9.

Hospital for Sick Children (1876) *Annual Report*, p. 1. HSC Archives, Toronto.

Hospital for Sick Children (1928) *Rules and Regulations*. HSC Archives, Toronto.

Hospital for Sick Children (1948) *Rules and Regulations*. HSC Archives, Toronto.

Hospital for Sick Children (1953, December 9) *Minutes of the Medical Advisory Board*. HSC Library, Toronto.

Hospital for Sick Children (1957, November 13). *Minutes of the Medical Advisory Board*. HSC Library, Toronto.

Hospital for Sick Children (1958, October) *Minutes of the Medical Advisory Board*. HSC Library, Toronto.

Hospital for Sick Children (1961, September) *Minutes of the Medical Advisory Board*. HSC Library, Toronto.

How to help your child prepare for hospital (1956, April 28). *Maclean's Magazine*. Scrapbook, HSC Archives, Toronto.

James, C.F. (1956) The parent's point of view. *Canadian Nurse*, **52**, 963–6.

Lamb, S. & Solomon, D.N. (1965) *The Social Behaviour Surrounding Children's Health Problems*. The Canadian Conference on Children, Ottawa.

MacDonald, M. (1969) Parents' participation in the care of the hospitalized child. *Canadian Nurse*, **65**(12), 37–9.

Meadows, S.R. (1969) The captive mother. *Archives of Disease in Childhood*, **44**, 362–7.

Ministry of Health (1959) *Platt Report on the Welfare of Children in Hospital*. Her Majesty's Stationery Office, London.

Mitchell, G. (1968) A child's response to consistent care. *Canadian Nurse*, **64**(9), 45–8.

New private wing opens at HSC (1935, June 12). *Toronto Telegram*. Scrapbook, HSC Archives, Toronto.

Prugh, D.G., Staub, E.M. & Sands, H.H. (1953) A study of the emotional reactions of children and families to hospitalization and illness. *American Journal of Orthopsychiatry*, **32**, 70– 106.

Robertson, J. (1953) Some responses of young children to loss of maternal care. *Nursing Times*, **49**, 382–6.

Robertson, J. (1970) *Young Children in Hospital*, 2nd edn. Cambridge University Press, Cambridge.

Rolstin, H. (1972) *The Hospital for Sick Children, Toronto: History of the School of Nursing*, p. 86. Charters, Toronto.

Rosenberg, C.E. (1987) *The Care of Strangers*, pp. 15–46. Basic Books, New York.

Spence, J. (1951) The doctor, the nurse and the sick child. *Canadian Nurse*, **47**, 13–16.

Spitz, R. (1945) Hospitalism. *Psychoanalytic Study of the Child*, **1**, 53–74.

Spock, B. (1946) *The Commonsense Book of Baby and Child Care*, pp. 25–6. Duell, Sloan & Pearce, New York.

Spock, B. (1957) *Baby and Child Care*, p.47. Meredith Press, New York.

Starr, P. (1982) *The Social Transformation of American Medicine*, pp. 145–79. Basic Books, New York.

Strong-Boag, V. (1976) Intruders in the nursery: child care professionals reshape the years one to five, 1920–1940. In *Childhood and Family in Canadian History* (ed. J. Parr), pp. 160–79. McClelland & Stewart, Toronto.

Vernon, D.T.A., Foley, J.M. & Sipowitz, R.R. (1965) *The Psychological Responses of Children to Hospitalization and Illness*. Thomas, Springfield, Illinois.

Vogel, M.J. (1980) *The Invention of the Modern Hospital*, p. 24. University of Chicago Press, Chicago.

Women's groups adopt projects for 1952 (1952, January 1). *Toronto Globe and Mail.* Scrapbook, HSC Archives, Toronto.

Young, J. (1987) Attitudes and practices towards the families of inpatients at the Hospital for Sick Children Toronto from 1935 to 1975. Unpublished master's thesis. Faculty of Nursing, University of Toronto, Ontario.

Young, J. (1990) Women founders, nurses and the care of children at the Hospital for Sick Children in Toronto 1875–99. In *Florence Nightingale and Her Era: A Collection of New Scholarship* (eds. V. Bullough, B. Bullough & M.P. Stanton), pp. 309–22. Garland, New York.

Young, J. (1992) A necessary nuisance: social class and parental visiting rights at Toronto's Hospital for Sick Children 1930–70. In *Canadian Health Care and the State* (ed. D. Naylor), pp. 85–103. McGill-Queen's University Press, Montreal and Kingston.

Your child in hospital (1952, April). *Toronto Star Weekly.* Scrapbook, HSC Archives, Toronto.

# Chapter 5
# Qualified nurses' perceptions of the needs of suddenly bereaved family members in the accident and emergency department

CHRISTOPHER TYE, BSc (Hons), RGN, RMN

Specialist Nurse Teacher (Accident and Emergency Nursing), Epsom and Kingston
College of Nursing and Midwifery, Epsom, Surrey, England

This study aimed to identify qualified nurses' perceptions of the
helpfulness of selected nursing actions, derived from the literature,
in meeting the needs of suddenly bereaved family members in the
accident and emergency (A&E) department. The effect of age, length
of professional experience and death education received on the
respondents' perceptions was examined. The nurse subjects' feelings
of preparation for this stressful role were also identified. A self-
administered, structured questionnaire using a five-point, Likert-
type rating scale and two open-ended questions was developed. A
non-randomized, convenience sample of 52 qualified nurses working
in three A&E departments in England's Greater London area was
used. Analysis of the sample's responses to the 35 nursing actions
included revealed that certain activities were ranked lower in terms
of their perceived helpfulness, compared to the survivors' perceptions in other studies. All three variables considered had a statistically significant correlation with the perceptions of the sample as
measured by the instrument ($P < 0.05$, using Mann-Whitney U-
test). Only 42% of the sample had received any form of death
education and 56% felt unprepared for this specialist role.

## Introduction

Whilst any bereavement represents a major emotional crisis, there is evidence
in the literature that sudden and unanticipated loss can be particularly
disabling (Lindemann, 1944; Bowlby, 1981; Lundin, 1984; Murphy, 1988;
Wright, 1991). Furthermore, the time immediately surrounding the death of
a close family member is considered to be crucial in determining a family's
ability to accept the death and to deal with the crisis (Dubin & Sarnoff, 1986;
Fraser & Atkins 1990).

Qualified nurses working in the accident and emergency (A&E) department inevitably encounter suddenly bereaved family members during the course of their professional work. It is therefore essential that A&E nurses should be adequately prepared to anticipate and meet the needs of this particular group, in order to facilitate the grieving process. As Worden (1982) highlights, 'Immobilised by the shock of the event, these families may not be able to ask for help and what they need'.

However, there are some indications that the needs of suddenly bereaved family members in the hospital setting are not always identified or met (Fanslow, 1983; Hill, 1988; Silvey, 1990; Finlay & Dallimore, 1991). Furthermore, the author's own experience of working in A&E departments has suggested that some nurses are not adequately prepared for this complex role and consequently may not always be aware of the needs of this particular group at a time of great crisis.

## The study

The aims of this study were:

(1) To establish what perceptions a sample of qualified nurses had of the helpfulness of a number of nursing actions, derived from the literature, in meeting the needs of suddenly bereaved family members in the A&E department.
(2) To identify whether the variables of age, length of professional experience in A&E nursing and death education received had a statistically significant correlation at the 0.05 level, with the perceptions of the sample as measured by the instrument used.
(3) To determine whether the sample of A&E nurses felt adequately prepared to undertake the stressful role of caring for suddenly bereaved family members.

## Literature review

### Sudden death

'When a sudden death occurs, families are faced with the enormous task of dealing with the loss of a significant relationship without preparation or warning' (Mian, 1990). Parkes (1975) identified a number of determinants of grief, which attempted to explain the differences between individuals in their response to bereavement. The mode of death, and in particular whether it was anticipated or sudden, was highlighted as one of the major factors influencing longer-term outcome.

Lundin (1984) found a significantly higher rate of morbidity during the first two years amongst individuals who had suffered a sudden loss, compared to those who expected the death. The lack of opportunity for family members to conceptualize the death is viewed by Williams (1984) as a major contributory factor to the additional stress of sudden bereavement. Without experiencing anticipatory grief, the shock is inevitably intense and numbing (Bowlby, 1981; Mian, 1990). The initial contact made with family members following the sudden death of a loved one, therefore, requires considerable psychosocial skills and knowledge of the grief process.

## Crisis theory

A sudden death that is unexpected represents an immensely stressful event in the survivor's life. The stress and emotional disturbance precipitated by the loss creates a crisis state (Schultz, 1980). Crisis is defined by Caplan (1964) as 'an upset or disequilibrium in a steady state occurring when usual problem solving strategies are ineffective'. These problem-solving strategies, or coping processes, are seen as psychological, self-regulatory mechanisms that, when used by the individual facilitate a return to homeostatic balance (Burgess & Baldwin, 1981). When an individual experiences such an emotionally hazardous situation and is unable to utilize previously learned coping behaviours effectively, or to reduce the stress using new, problem-solving strategies, an emotional crisis may ensue.

Extreme stressors, such as the sudden, unexpected death of a spouse, commonly impair the survivor's ability to cope in the short-term and may lead to longer-term psychological disturbance. The individual in crisis perceives a state of upset, an uncertainty of outcome and feelings of helplessness (Graves 1984). As the crisis progresses, increasing tension and other varied physiological manifestations lead to decreased function levels. Immediately following a crisis event, prompt and skilful interventions are necessary to assist individuals towards maintaining or regaining emotional equilibrium (Murgatroyd & Woolfe, 1982; Woolley, 1990).

Crisis Intervention is based on the assumption that specific behaviour patterns can be directly related to certain kinds of crisis events (Aguilera & Messick, 1986). The first stage of crisis intervention following sudden bereavement consists of an appraisal or assessment of the situation based upon the expected behaviour patterns specific to this type of crisis event. A decision must then be made on the type of help required. Skilled intervention should be designed to promote adaptation and regain equilibrium (Woolley, 1990).

It is apparent, therefore, that following the crisis of sudden death, which frequently renders the survivor unable to formulate coping strategies, skilful nursing interventions based on a knowledge of the grieving process and the identified needs of these individuals may help to facilitate positive long-term outcomes.

### Suddenly bereaved family members in the A&E department

A qualitative study, based in Leeds General Infirmary A&E department, England, attempted to explore the survivors' perceptions of their immediate care following the sudden loss of a loved one (Ashdown, 1985). The relatives' room used to accommodate suddenly bereaved families was widely criticized as being unsuitably positioned and lacking natural light.

None of the sample described feelings of regret at viewing the body. The importance of confirming the reality of the situation in order to set people free from their worse fears of what might have happened, was also well illustrated.

Some unfavourable comments were made about the containers that were used to return property. Medical staff, who spent only brief periods with the relatives, were also criticized by a number of subjects, who felt they lacked sensitivity and interpersonal skills. The way the news of death was communicated appeared to have long-term effects, and the survivors were able to recall with remarkable clarity particular words used.

In the United States there have been a number of studies which provide useful insights into the survivors' perceptions of their immediate needs and the nursing interventions which were seen as helpful or unhelpful in coping with the disabling impact of sudden death (Jones & Buttery, 1981; Williams, 1984; Mian, 1990; Fraser & Atkins, 1990). The frequency with which similar interventions appear elsewhere in the literature (Fanslow, 1983; Dubin & Sarnoff, 1986; Hadfield, 1987; McLauchlan, 1990; Yates *et al.*, 1990) further reinforces the importance of certain actions in facilitating the early grief process.

### Preparation and training for nurses

In attempting to examine the needs of suddenly bereaved family members, several of the above studies have indicated that there is considerable room for improvement in the skills used by some health care professionals (Jones & Buttery, 1981; Yates *et al.*, 1990).

In addition, a survey by Finlay & Dallimore (1991) into the views of parents on how the death of their children was handled revealed a number of disturbing findings. For example, 34 of the 120 respondents rated the interview when news of death was broken as badly handled or offensive. Also, the police were rated as being more sympathetic than the nurses or doctors, which the authors suggested might be due to the inclusion of some teaching on breaking bad news in police training.

The lack of relevant education for nurses in the area of sudden death is highlighted by several authors (Field & Kitson, 1986; McGuinness, 1988; Sherr, 1989; Eastham, 1990; Cooke *et al.*, 1992), implying that many nurses are not adequately prepared for this stressful role. In the absence of training programmes, many A&E nurses 'learn' through repeated exposure to sudden death events, often without the benefit of any subsequent feedback on their interventions. Thus bad skills can become entrenched and difficult to 'unlearn' (Sherr, 1989).

**Summary of literature review**

A review of the literature has indicated the crisis nature of sudden unanticipated loss. A number of American studies have aimed to determine the survivors' perceptions of their emergency department experience following the sudden death of a loved one. There would appear to be a number of nursing interventions identified in these studies and elsewhere, which are described as helpful in meeting the needs of this particular group. However, there is some evidence that this crucial period at the very beginning of the grieving process is not always managed in a sensitive or skilled manner.

The central role of the qualified nurse in the A&E department when confronted with suddenly bereaved family members is widely recognized. However, it is claimed that many lack training in grief counselling and consequently feel inadequately prepared to meet the immediate needs of the survivors. This study, therefore, aimed to bring together the above elements in a United Kingdom setting, using a sample of qualified nurses working in three different A&E departments.

## Methodology

The method selected for this study was an exploratory, descriptive sample survey utilizing a structured, self-administered questionnaire designed by the author. In order to gather data from the nurse subjects in a form that would allow responses to be standardized and statistically analysed, a primarily quantitative approach was taken. However, since the subject area was potentially sensitive, some qualitative data were collected to add supplementary depth and colour to the study.

**Development of the questionnaire**

It was first necessary to identify from the literature a suitably comprehensive list of nursing activities relevant to this time of crisis. As indicated above, Fraser & Atkins' (1990) study aimed to discover the survivors' recollections of helpful and unhelpful emergency nurse activities which the authors had derived from the literature. The study used 'an investigator constructed' questionnaire containing 18 nurse activities.

A number of other studies were used to modify and supplement Fraser & Atkins' (1990) list, creating a final total of 35 actions. In order to ensure a logical structure, the nursing actions were organized into a series of phases which were intended to reflect the family members' A&E department experience.

A total of nine phases were identified and incorporated in the instrument as follows:

(1) Contacting the family members and dealing with them promptly on arrival.
(2) Providing suitable private facilities.
(3) Providing one nurse to act as liaison between the family members and resuscitation team.
(4) Providing information about the severity of the patient's condition prior to death and preparing the family for the possibility that death may ensue.
(5) Breaking the news of death.
(6) Viewing the body and respecting religious customs following death.
(7) Dealing with the grief reaction of the family members and the emotional response of the staff involved.
(8) Providing information about the cause of death, postmortem examinations and what to do next.
(9) Providing follow-up arrangements from the department and concluding the process.

A five-point Likert-type rating scale of 'not helpful; slightly helpful; moderately helpful; very helpful and one of the most helpful' was used to provide a sufficient range of options. Each nurse subject was asked to place 'one tick only' for every nursing action, on the point of the scale of helpfulness which they felt was appropriate. In order to minimize potential response set bias, it was emphasized that there were 'no right or wrong answers' and that each nursing action should be considered individually.

An open question asking respondents to comment, if they wished, on any of the nursing actions was included. Demographic data requested were gender, age, nursing qualifications, current position/title and length of experience in A&E nursing.

The final section of the instrument asked respondents whether they had received any formal education or training in dealing with bereavement and whether they felt adequately prepared to meet the needs of suddenly bereaved family members.

A small pilot study was carried out using six qualified nurses on a post-basic A&E nursing course. As a result, some minor alterations were made to the spacing and layout of the questionnaire.

**Reliability and validity**

The internal consistency of the instrument was measured using a split-half test (Pearson $r = 0.699$). Because the 35 nursing actions used in the questionnaire were derived from an extensive search of the literature, which provided a range of corroborative sources, a degree of content validity could be claimed. Calling upon expert opinion is regarded as a further measure of the potential representativeness of the content area (Polit & Hungler, 1989). The instrument was therefore shown to several senior A&E nursing specialists and Macmillan nurse tutors prior to the main study and appropriate modifications were made.

**Sample**

In order to obtain a sample of reasonable size, three different general hospitals in the Greater London area in England were selected. A non-randomized sample of convenience, consisting of all the qualified A&E nursing staff employed at the time of the study, was used ($n = 70$). It was hoped to reduce response set bias by using a number of different hospitals, where the nursing 'culture' might vary.

Of the 70 questionnaires sent out, 52 were adequately completed and returned, representing a response rate of 74%.

*Data analysis and findings*

Although the sample contained a wide range of age, experience and grades (Table 5.1), over half (58%) had never received any form of training. Furthermore, only seven (13%) indicated they had received education in this area during basic nurse training. Ten of the sample (19%) stated that they had received training in dealing with suddenly bereaved relatives during the ENBCNS 199 (Accident and Emergency Nursing) course, and 10 (19%) had attended study days on, for example, breaking bad news.

**Perceptions of the helpfulness of nursing actions**

The subjects' scores (1–5) for each nursing action were totalled and put in rank order, the highest score representing the action which the sample as a whole thought was the most helpful in meeting the needs of suddenly

**Table 5.1**  Demographic data of sample.

| Variable | Number of subjects ($n = 52$) | % |
|---|---|---|
| A.  Sex | | |
| Male | 4 | 8 |
| Female | 48 | 92 |
| B.  Age | | |
| 21–30 | 28 | 54 |
| 31–40 | 19 | 36 |
| 41–50 | 3 | 6 |
| 51+ | 2 | 4 |
| C.  Nursing qualification | | |
| Enrolled nurse | 8 | 15 |
| Registered nurse | 44 | 85 |
| D.  Current position/title | | |
| Enrolled nurse | 6 | 12 |
| Senior enrolled nurse | 2 | 4 |
| Staff nurse | 25 | 48 |
| Senior staff nurse | 9 | 17 |
| Sister/charge nurse | 10 | 19 |
| E.  Length of experience in A&E nursing | | |
| < 1 year | 12 | 23 |
| 1–5 years | 18 | 35 |
| > 5 years | 22 | 42 |

bereaved family members, and the lowest score being the least helpful (Table 5.2). The range of scores calculated was 97–239.

The action which this sample of nurse subjects felt was the most helpful was number 2, 'dealing with the family promptly on arrival in the department'. The second most helpful action, 'providing a room for the use of the family', was ranked by Fraser & Atkins' (1990) sample of survivors as the most helpful action, indicating a degree of congruence across the groups. It should be noted, however, that direct comparison is problematic owing to differences in the instruments used.

Nursing action 4, 'providing comfort measures such as tea or coffee', was ranked 22nd in terms of its perceived helpfulness. However, other studies have indicated that family members greatly appreciate these sorts of basic comfort measures (Ashdown, 1985; Fraser & Atkins, 1990; Mian, 1990).

'Providing information about the treatment given prior to death' (action 8) was ranked relatively low by the sample of nurses in this study (26th). This was interesting in the light of the growing debate surrounding family members' presence during resuscitation. Whilst the American experience in one emergency centre appears positively evaluated by the relatives (Hansen &

**Table 5.2**  Rank order of total scores of individual nursing actions for whole sample ($n$ = 52) (adapted from Fraser & Atkins (1990), with permission of Mosby-Year Book, Inc., St Louis)

| Rank order | Nursing action | Questionnaire number | Total score |
|---|---|---|---|
| (1) | Dealing with the family promptly on arrival | 2 | 239 |
| (2) | Providing a separate room for the use of the family | 3 | 233 |
| (2) | Allowing time to listen to grieving family members | 23 | 233 |
| (4) | Identifying one nurse to remain with the family throughout stay | 5 | 231 |
| (5) | Allowing family to talk about their anxieties | 10 | 229 |
| (6) | Giving permission to the family to touch or hold the body | 20 | 228 |
| (6) | Respecting different customs following death | 25 | 228 |
| (8) | Providing written information about what to do following a death | 31 | 227 |
| (9) | Offering emotional support to the family | 14 | 223 |
| (10) | Giving information about the severity of the patient's condition as early as possible | 7 | 222 |
| (11) | Showing concern and caring to the family about the death | 13 | 219 |
| (11) | Ensuring family members do not go home alone | 30 | 219 |
| (13) | Preparing the family for the possibility that death may ensue | 9 | 216 |
| (14) | Encouraging full expression of grief | 22 | 215 |
| (14) | Ensuring that the family have clearly understood the news of death | 12 | 215 |
| (16) | Preparing the family for what to expect before viewing the body | 17 | 214 |
| (16) | Providing an outside telephone line | 6 | 214 |
| (18) | Removing any unnecessary equipment from the body prior to viewing | 18 | 208 |
| (19) | If contacting by telephone, giving the family member a name to ask for on arrival in the department | 1 | 205 |
| (20) | Allowing the family to phone a named person in the department if they require further information | 33 | 201 |
| (21) | Giving the opportunity to ask about the cause of death, if known | 27 | 196 |
| (22) | Providing comfort measures, such as tea or coffee | 4 | 194 |
| (23) | Allowing viewing of the body in the department | 15 | 193 |
| (24) | Discouraging feelings of guilt about the death | 24 | 190 |
| (24) | Staying with the family member whilst viewing the body | 19 | 190 |
| (26) | Providing information about the treatment given prior to death | 8 | 184 |
| (27) | Explaining about postmortem examinations, if applicable | 28 | 171 |
| (28) | Giving information about 'normal' grief symptoms | 29 | 167 |
| (29) | Showing your own emotional response to the death | 21 | 163 |
| (30) | Indicating to the family when it is OK to leave the department | 35 | 161 |
| (31) | Ensuring a doctor breaks the news of death | 11 | 152 |
| (32) | Providing a follow-up phone call from the department after a few weeks | 32 | 132 |
| (33) | Ensuring all clothing is returned to the family regardless of its condition | 34 | 126 |
| (34) | Offering sedation to family members | 26 | 105 |
| (35) | Discouraging viewing of the body if seriously mutilated | 16 | 97 |

Strawser, 1992), the issue remains controversial in the United Kingdom. Skilful facilitation and sensitive management on an individual basis, are clearly key requirements for successful implementation.

'Allowing viewing of the body in the department' (action 15) was ranked 23rd in this study. This appeared to be in contrast to the importance attached to providing immediate confirmation of the death, identified by family members elsewhere in the literature (Jones & Buttery, 1981; Cathcart, 1988; Mian, 1990; Scowen, 1990). However, other aspects of viewing the body included in the instrument attracted higher scores, which suggested that the location of viewing was perceived as the key issue. For example, the clinical environment of the resuscitation room may have been regarded as unsuitable in this context by some of the respondents, with the associated pressures of lack of time and space for other emergency care. This contrasts however with Wright's (1991) view that it is important for family members to see their loved one where they died, rather than in another separate area such as a chapel of rest.

*Emotional response to death*

Nursing action 21, 'showing your own emotional response to the death', was ranked 29th. There appeared to be an unwillingness amongst some of the sample to express personal emotions in this situation. Yet Finlay & Dallimore's (1991) study of suddenly bereaved parents concluded:

'Parents gained great support from being aware that the informant was also upset – for example, "he cared so much he had tears in his eyes", whereas the colder, businesslike informant tended to cause great offence.'

Parkes (1975) also claims that a willingness to reveal personal feelings by the professional shows the relatives they are not ashamed of these feelings or rendered useless by them.

Several of the nursing actions concerned with follow-up (e.g. number 32, 'providing a follow-up phone call from the department after a few weeks') were ranked low in terms of their perceived helpfulness. This area appears to have been developed to a far greater extent in the United States, whereas traditionally in England follow-up has not been seen as part of the A&E nurse's role. Yet, there is evidence which appears to indicate how useful some surviving family members can find talking to a health care professional who was actually present at the time of death, or who was involved with them when the news of death was broken (Mian, 1990).

In contrast to this view, several nurse respondents indicated by their comments that they felt this might be an intrusion, or painful reminder:

'A follow-up phone call at home may intrude on private grief.'

'I feel phoning after a few weeks may bring it all home to the family and may not be helpful.'

The sample of nurses in the study felt overall that 'ensuring a doctor breaks the news of death' was not helpful, relative to the other actions (31st). This was further reinforced by several of the respondent's comments:

'My experience of doctors breaking bad news is that they are very bad at it and often do not make it clear that the patient has died.'

'I think it is completely unnecessary for doctors to break news – [it] should be the person who has had the most dealings with them.'

Historically, many doctors have seen this area as their sole responsibility, and it remains important for the survivors to have medical questions answered properly, if required. However, the way the news is broken and the interpersonal skills used in this situation vastly outweigh professional role demarcation.

Offering sedation was also ranked very low (34th) which is supported by the literature, as it may seriously interfere with, or suppress altogether, the grieving process (Hill, 1988; Wright, 1991).

### Perceptions of helpfulness in relation to age, length of professional experience and death education received

In order to analyse this aspect of the study, each nurse subject's total score was calculated for all 35 nursing actions. The possible range of total scores was thus 35–175. Having calculated each subject's total score, the sample was divided up according to the variable under consideration: age, length of professional experience and death education received. Personal variables such as these are often claimed to have a correlation with individual perceptions and attitudes (Treece & Treece, 1986).

The two sets of scores for each of the variables were then analysed using a Mann–Whitney U-test. The results indicated that all three variables under consideration had a statistically significant correlation with the ranking of the nurse subjects' perceptions of helpfulness as measured by the instrument used ($P < 0.05$). As the level of significance accepted for the study was 0.05, the null hypothesis that there would be no significant difference in the perceptions of the sample in relation to the variables of age, length of A&E experience and death education received was rejected in each case.

Whilst education has been shown to have a correlation with nurses' perceptions, as suggested by Miles (1980) and Lyons (1988), age (which could be equated with 'life experience') and length of specialist professional experience appeared to be equally important factors in this particular study.

**Perceptions of preparedness**

Over half the sample (56%) felt they were not adequately prepared for this role, despite having to manage such crisis situations on a recurring basis. This finding agrees with McGuiness' (1988) study, where 50% of the sample surveyed felt inadequately prepared. Of the 29 respondents who did not feel adequately prepared, 20 (69%) had not received any formal death education and 23 (79%) had less than five years A&E nursing experience.

The perceived value of training *and* experience in preparing nurses for this role was also well illustrated by some of the respondents' comments:

'I am certain I would benefit from any further training, and although I learnt from trial and error, I do not feel that new or junior staff should have to do the same.'

'I think I cope well with most situations. I must stress that I have only gained this through years of experience and would have appreciated more training in this field.'

Also the stress imposed on nurses involved in sudden bereavement was made apparent. For example:

'It is a situation where I feel uncomfortable, upset. I find it difficult to speak to relatives in this situation, being frightened of upsetting them further.'

## *Discussion*

The sample of 52 qualified nurses used in this study appeared overall to have a reasonable level of awareness of the needs of suddenly bereaved family members, as measured by the instrument used. However, within the sample there were a variety of differing perceptions of the helpfulness of individual actions.

The sample as a whole indicated that certain actions, such as 'offering sedation to family members', 'ensuring a doctor breaks the news of death' and 'returning all clothing to the family regardless of its condition', were not perceived as helpful in this situation. This is supported, in the main, by other studies which have sought the survivors' opinions. However, certain actions which have been identified as very helpful elsewhere, such as 'providing comfort measures' (Fraser & Atkins, 1990) and 'allowing viewing of the body in the department' (Mian, 1990) were ranked much lower in terms of their helpfulness by this sample of nurses.

In addition, the sample as a whole perceived that follow-up services in the A&E department were not particularly helpful. This contradicts current practice in many emergency departments in the United States, as well as certain centres in the UK (Yates *et al.*, 1990; Cooke *et al.*, 1992). The study also found that over half of the sample had not received any death education, either at basic or post-registration level. This finding is, perhaps, disturbing in the light of many authors in this field who claim that training is a crucial component in the effective management of sudden bereavement (e.g. Lyons, 1988; Sherr, 1989; Wright, 1991).

Age, length of specialist experience and death education received were all shown to have a statistically significant correlation with the perceptions of the nurse subjects regarding the needs of family members immediately following sudden bereavement ($P < 0.05$). The limitations of the instrument and the non-randomized sample used prohibit any generalizable conclusions to be drawn from this. However, education alone does not appear to be sufficient preparation in this context. Equally, experience without some form of preparation or evaluation seems unsatisfactory. The lack of comparable studies in this specific area of sudden death makes reference to other work impossible.

## Sensitivity and self-awareness

However, the literature does indicate that sensitivity, self-awareness and flexibility are important qualities in the professionals involved (Penson, 1990; McLauchlan, 1990).

Recognizing the validity of the carer's own emotional reaction to the tragedy was also highlighted by the sample's responses to this particular action in the questionnaire. The apparent unwillingness of the sample to reveal their own feelings may represent an attempt to avoid or withdraw from the pain associated with sudden loss (Johansson & Lally, 1990). As such, it could be viewed as a defence against the threat of repeated exposure to highly intense emotional experiences (Holman, 1990).

The study also revealed that under half of the sample felt adequately prepared for their role in managing sudden bereavement. Again, the results suggested that training *and* experience were both essential elements in feeling adequately prepared. However, it remains questionable whether feeling prepared for this difficult role necessarily leads to nurses making more effective interventions with the survivors in sudden death crises. Equally, awareness of the range of nursing interventions which might be helpful to the survivors does not automatically translate into good nursing practice in the clinical environment.

## *Implications for nursing practice/education*

Many of the nursing actions identified from the literature as helpful and included in the instrument could form the basis of a sudden bereavement intervention tool for use in the A&E department setting. Similar tools have already been used successfully in the United States and have proved to be useful frameworks for educational purposes. It must be emphasized that such a tool should only be used as a guide for assessment and not rigidly applied regardless of the situation or individuals concerned.

The lack of educational or training opportunities found in the study and the number of nurses who felt inadequately prepared should be a cause for concern. Whilst other aspects of the study indicated that training was not the only variable that had an effect on perceptions, it is clearly an important element, particularly in less experienced staff. Equally, it should be recognized that experienced staff need the opportunity to reflect on and review their clinical practice.

It is recommended that any training provided should be relevant to the particular needs of the suddenly bereaved, and should concentrate on psychosocial and interpersonal skills. Self-awareness and personal attitudes towards death and dying should also be explored experientially, as suggested by Durlak & Riesenberg (1991). Doctors, as well as nurses, need to be involved. Most importantly, whenever possible the training provided should draw on and develop the clinical experiences of the staff concerned.

Along with this, attention needs to be given to who should break the news of death. The historical monopoly of the medical profession in this area has already been challenged in some centres. Whoever carries out this role must possess the necessary skills and sensitivity, as well as having had some previous contact with the survivors during their time in the department.

Consideration should also be given to developing some form of follow-up service from the A&E department in order to provide continuing support in the community.

Finally, the mere fact that there is so little research into this area, especially in the United Kingdom, underlines the need for further work. The few studies that are available indicate that much remains to be done if the needs of this vulnerable group are to be met during their brief stay in the A&E department and beyond.

## References

Aguilera, D.C. & Messick, J.M. (1986) *Crisis Intervention – Theory and Methodology*, 5th edn. C.V. Mosby, St. Louis.

Ashdown, M. (1985) Sudden death. *Nursing Mirror*, **161**(18). 22–4.

Bowlby, J. (1981) *Loss, Sadness and Depression*. Penguin, Harmondsworth, Middlesex.

Burgess, A.W. & Baldwin, B.A. (1981) *Crisis Intervention: Theory and Practice*. Prentice Hall, Englewood Cliffs, New Jersey.

Caplan, G. (1964) *Principles of Preventative Psychiatry*. Basic Books, New York.

Cathcart, F. (1988) Seeing the body after death. *British Medical Journal*, **297**, 997–8.

Cooke, M.W., Cooke, H.M. & Glucksman, E.E. (1992) Management of sudden bereavement in the accident and emergency department. *British Medical Journal*, **304**, 1207–9.

Dubin, W.R. & Sarnoff, J.R. (1986) Sudden and unexpected death: intervention with the survivors. *Annals of Emergency Medicine*, **15**(1), 54–7.

Durlak, J.A. & Riesenberg, L.A. (1991) The impact of death education. *Death Studies*, **15**(1), 39–58.

Eastham, K. (1990) Dealing with bereavement in critical care. *Intensive Care Nursing*, **6**, 185–91.

Fanslow, J. (1983) Needs of grieving spouses in sudden death situations: a pilot study. *Journal of Emergency Nursing*, **9**(4), 213–17.

Field, D. & Kitson, C. (1986) Formal teaching about death and dying in nursing schools. *Nurse Education*, **6**, 270–6.

Finlay, I. & Dallimore, D. (1991) Your child is dead. *British Medical Journal*, **302**, 1524–5.

Fraser, S. & Atkins, J. (1990) Survivor's recollections of helpful and unhelpful emergency nurse activities surrounding the sudden death of a loved one. *Journal of Emergency Nursing*, **16**(1), 13–16.

Graves, P. (1984) Intervening in crisis. In *Community Health: Nursing Process and Procedure for Promoting Health* (eds M. Stanhope & J. Lancaster), pp. 432–44. C.V. Mosby, New York.

Hadfield, L. (1987) Caring for the suddenly bereaved in the A and E department. *Emergency Nurse*, **2**(1), 3–4.

Hansen, C. & Strawser, D. (1992) Family presence during cardiopulmonary resuscitation: Foote Hospital Emergency Department's nine year perspective. *Journal of Emergency Nursing*, **18**(2), 104–6.

Hill, J. (1988) Bereavement care. In *Nursing Issues and Research in Terminal Care* (eds J. Wilson-Barnett & J. Raiman), pp. 37–53. J. Wiley and Sons, Chichester.

Holman, E.A. (1990) Death and the health professional. Organisation and defence in health care. *Death Studies*, **14**(1), 13–24.

Johansson, N. & Lally, T. (1990) Effectiveness of a death education programme in reducing death anxiety of nursing students. *Omega Journal of Death and Dying*, **22**(1), 25–33.

Jones, W.H. & Buttery, M. (1981) Sudden death: survivors' perceptions of the emergency department experience. *Journal of Emergency Nursing*, **7**(1), 14–17.

Lindemann, E. (1944) Symptomatology and management of acute grief. *American Journal of Psychiatry*, **101**, 141–9.

Lundin, T. (1984) Long-term outcome of bereavement. *British Journal of Psychiatry*, **145**, 424–8.

Lyons, J. (1988) Bereavement and death education: a survey of nurses' views. *Nurse Education Today*, **8**, 168–72.

McGuinness, S. (1988) Sudden death in the emergency department. In *Management and Practice in Emergency Nursing* (ed. B. Wright), pp. 133–64. Chapman and Hall, London.

McLauchlan, C.A.J. (1990) Handling distressed relatives and breaking bad news. *British Medical Journal*, **301**, 1145–9.

Mian, P. (1990) Sudden bereavement: nursing interventions in the E.D. *Critical Care Nurse*, **10**(1), 30–40.

Miles, M.S. (1980) The effect of a course on death and grief on nurses' attitudes towards dying patients and death. *Death Education*, **4**, 245–60.

Murgatroyd, S. & Woolfe, R. (1982) *Coping with Crisis, Understanding and Helping People in Need*. Harper and Row, London.

Murphy, S.A. (1988) Mental distress and recovery in a high-risk bereavement sample three years after untimely death. *Nursing Research*, **37**(1), 30–5.

Parkes, C.M. (1975) *Bereavement: Studies of Grief in Adult Life*. Pelican, Harmondsworth, Middlesex.

Penson, J. (1990) *Bereavement: A Guide for Nurses*. Harper and Row, London.

Polit, D.F. & Hungler, B.P. (1989) *Essentials of Nursing Research: Methods, Appraisal and Utilisation*, 2nd edn. J.B. Lipincott, Philadelphia.

Schultz, C.A. (1980) Sudden death crisis: pre-hospital and in the emergency department. *Journal of Emergency Nursing*, **6**(3), 46–50.

Scowen, P. (1990) Viewing the body after death. *Bereavement Care*, **9**(3), 35–6.

Sherr, L. (1989) Staff training: a necessity not a luxury. In *Death, Dying and Bereavement* (ed. L. Sherr), pp. 48–68. Blackwell Scientific Publications, Oxford.

Silvey, S. (1990) Bereavement care in hospitals. *Bereavement Care*, **9**(2), 17–18.

Treece, E. & Treece, J. (1986) *Elements of Research in Nursing*, 4th edn. C.V. Mosby, St Louis.

Williams, M. (1984) Use of a concluding process to assist grieving families. *Journal of Emergency Nursing*, **10**(5), 254–8.

Woolley, N. (1990) Crisis theory: a paradigm of effective intervention with families of critically ill people. *Journal of Advanced Nursing*, **15**, 1402–8.

Worden, J.W. (1982). *Grief Counselling and Grief Therapy*. Springer, New York.

Wright, B. (1991) *Sudden Death: Intervention Skills for the Caring Professions*. Churchill Livingstone, Edinburgh.

Yates, D.W., Ellison, G. & McGuinness, S. (1990) Care of the suddenly bereaved. *British Medical Journal*, **301**, 29–31.

# Chapter 6
# The experience of a community characterized by violence: a challenge for nursing

EDITH NONHLANHLA MADELA, *RN, MCur*
D.Cur (Psychiatric Nursing) Candidate, Rand Afrikaans University

and MARIE POGGENPOEL, *RN, DPhil*
Professor of Nursing, Department of Nursing Science, Rand Afrikaans University, Johannesburg, Transvaal, Republic of South Africa

Social situations make a person vulnerable to mental illness. These situations include circumstances such as poverty, family instability and inadequate nutrition. A combination of these circumstances predisposes exposed people to developing unhealthy ways of coping with stress. Violence is seen as a way of managing stress, but also as a factor causing stress. An example of unhealthy ways of stress management in the current South African society is the violence that leads to unrest which has affected different communities in a short space of time. The aim of this study was to explore the experience of a community exposed to violence and to identify implications for nursing. An exploratory contextual study was undertaken with the purpose of generating meaning regarding the experience of a community characterized by violence. The phenomenological method of interviewing was used to gather data. The target population consisted of a township community of 228 000. Ten respondents were interviewed in total, selected by the convenience purposive sampling method through intermediaries. The interviews were recorded on tape and later transcribed verbatim. Data were analysed by the method of content analysis. The results were centred on the respondents' and their families' experiences of violence since March 1990. The results indicated four types of experiences for all people exposed to violence: psychological, spiritual, physical and behavioural experiences. The experiences of interactions with the internal environment (psychological, spiritual and physical experience) were predominantly negative, except for only two positive spiritual experiences (improvements in the people's faith and in the employer–employee relationships). On the other hand, experiences of interactions between the internal and external environments, namely behavioural experiences, were both negative and positive. The negative experiences included pretence, thuggery, scapegoating and harassment. The positive experiences included solidarity, bravery and increased appreciation. The presence of positive experiences in both environments brought about new insights; that is, that even though most of their internal environment and part of their external environment is bleak and hopeless, the victims of violence still have the will to survive and live a normal life like other people. This positive attitude supplies the psychiatric nurse with a point of entry to bring about positive change that acts as a support for the community exposed to violence. Possibilities of applying the results of this study in education, practice and research in the health field became evident.

## Rationale and objectives of research

Health in Africa is viewed as a function of the community. It is an indigenous concept that acceptance within, and harmony with family and society are important elements of healing and preserving health of people (Atkins, 1984).

In line with this is the viewpoint that social situations make a person vulnerable to mental illness. These situations include circumstances such as poverty, family instability and inadequate nutrition. Deprivation throughout the life cycle leaves the individual with a limited ability to cope with stress, as the person has few available environmental support systems. This combination of circumstances leads the exposed person to a predisposition to develop unhealthy ways of coping with stress. Violence can be seen as a way of managing stress, but also as a factor causing stress (stressor). An example of unhealthy ways of stress management in present South African society is the violence that leads to unrest which has affected different communities within a short space of time (Anon., 1990a,b).

Conditions like an increase in theft and other social–pathological phenomena occur because personal lives of community members are threatened and there is the problem with accommodation, and electricity, water and sewerage are cut off (Burgers, 1990, Singh, 1990). This gives rise to an increase in unhealthy stress levels in members, and therefore makes them vulnerable to the development of mental illness (Stuart & Sudeen, 1987).

## Violence

In the community where Edith Madela's relatives have lived, for as long as she can remember, things were going as smoothly as in any so-called healthy community (Madela, 1991). However, after the onset of the violence that took place around March 1990, which was termed the most concentrated violence in South Africa since the Second World War (Grange, 1990), she observed a lot of changes in the functioning of the community. There was overall depression and the whole community suffered many problems.

Smith (1990) stated that there is a very real danger that all of us feel overwhelmed by the violence in our society and withdraw into a kind of survival mentality. This, she continued, involves an emotional anaesthesia, a disengagement from others, a retreat from social involvement into a private defensive core.

Vogelman (1990) conducted a study on workers in which he identified the hostel as a breeding ground or starting point for much of the violence. He identified prime difficulties that individuals face when living in a war zone, like transport and travel, and suggested that psychological counselling would help decrease some of the psychological difficulties arising from the violence.

Violence, together with the existing factors like inadequate housing, evictions, lack of sleep and money, long travelling hours and transport difficulties, affects the community in many ways. These effects can be divided into three main categories: spiritual, psychological and physical.

### Spiritual effects

Spiritual effects refers to all disturbances regarding values, ethical principles, meaning in life and relationships as reflected in: homicide, family dissolutions, vandalism, arson, terrorism, robbery, infanticide, child and woman abuse, familicide, divorce, unemployment, reduced school performance, poverty, militancy and low productivity (Grange, 1990; Singh, 1990; Smith, 1990).

### Psychological effects

Psychological effects refers to all intellectual, emotional and volitional effects including emotional anaesthesia, blunting of human sensibilities, mental illness, low school and work performance, a high level of stress, anxiety, fear and suspicion (Gibson, 1986; Lab 1988; Smith 1990).

### Physical effects

Physical effects refers to structural and functional effects in the community and includes damage to property, arson, poverty, unemployment and loss of property (Smith, 1990; Vogelman, 1990).

Thus, the black communities have suffered severe consequences of stress caused by violence as well as other factors mentioned above. To make matters worse, municipal councils cut electricity, water, sewerage and tele-phone systems (Anders & Hlophe, 1990). These conditions caused crises for many people and exposed them to an insecure, deprived environment.

## Silence of professionals

In 1979 the American Psychiatric Association released a statement based on the work of a panel of psychiatrists who were sent to South Africa. In it they pointed out the silence of local mental health professionals (Vogelman, 1986). Vogelman (1986) added that, to date, with few exceptions South Africans working within the mental health sphere have been slow to respond to the social context of deprivation, which is true of the black communities in South Africa.

As long ago as 1976, a work group of the WHO produced a report on the role of nursing in psychiatric and mental health care in which it stressed that the role should be developed and strengthened, especially primary health care (Poggenpoel, 1984). Thus, by becoming aware of these effects of an insecure, deprived environment, the psychiatric nurse must assess the effects of unhealthy coping mechanisms as reflected in violence, and plan and imple-ment supportive programmes for high-risk populations.

Based on these identified problems the primary goal of this research was:

(1) To explore the experience of individuals in a black community characterized by violence and based on the information gathered.
(2) To make recommendations regarding the implications of the results on nursing education, nursing practice and nursing research.

## *Research design and method*

This research study was an exploratory study with the purpose of increasing insight and generating meaning regarding the experience of stress by indi-viduals in a community characterized by violence (Burns & Grove, 1987; Mouton & Marais, 1989). The phenomenological method of interviewing was utilized to obtain data. It was a contextual study in that individuals in a specific community were studied (Mouton & Marais, 1989). It was a quali-tative study in that it was aimed at the best possible understanding of the experience of stress by individuals in a community characterized by violence (Madela, 1991).

The researchers gave attention to reliability and validity measures as described by Woods & Catanzaro (1988) while completing the research project.

## Reliability

Reliability measures employed to ensure the reliability of the method utilized in this research project included: clearly identifying the researcher's role as postgraduate psychiatric nursing student; describing the content and development of the researcher's role as the study evolved; encouraging intermediaries to recruit participants non-selectively; delineating the context (social, physical and interpersonal) in which data were generated; describing characteristics of participants and the decision processes involved in their choice to participate; taping the interviews to ensure accurate recall of the structure and function of the context; reporting precisely and thoroughly the strategies used to collect, analyse and code data; transcribing tape-recorded interviews verbatim; using at least two codes to perform theoretical coding; phrasing low inference inscriptors in concrete precise terms and comparing findings with published studies and other investigators pursuing similar work (Woods & Catanzaro, 1988).

## Validity

Validity measures employed to ensure validity of the method used included: identifying those changes that were recurrent, progressive and cyclical as the sources of change; distinguishing maturation from effects of interviewing phenomena by use of constant comparative analysis and discrepant case analysis; using independent corroboration from multiple participants, discrepant-case analysis and observation: utilizing substantive and theoretical coding likely to elicit contrived responses; comparing data to theories and analytical models derived from literature; presenting data in relation to researcher's position and relationship; constant comparative analysis and validity checks with participants, which the researcher did by playing back the tapes to participants, after taping the interview to verify the contents with them; questioning of commonly assumed meanings, and utilization of discrepant-case analysis; reminding participants often that they are experts in topic of study; provision of consistent follow-up to participants in the form of information about the ongoing study; making it easy for the participants to notify the researcher of their change of address by providing them with return postcards and giving them Edith Madela's relatives' full address, who live in the same township; and recruiting those participants who meet purposive sampling criteria (Woods & Catanzaro, 1988).

## Population

The target population for the research was selected from a specific black township on the Witwatersrand. It is a relatively small township with a population of 228 000 individuals. It is divided into five sections, each with five to eight streets, each street with seven to 18 houses, depending on the length of the street. The community consists of all ethnic groups. Individuals included in the research had to comply with the following criteria:

(1) They had to have been citizens of the township for at least two years, since the worst violence had started just over a year before.
(2) They had to have been there when violence broke out in March 1990 to have experienced its effects.
(3) They had to be heads of the families living in the houses included in the sample or equivalents thereof, irrespective of sex.
(4) They had to be between 18 and 70 years of age to have been able to appreciate the effects of the violence and to remember the details.
(5) They had to be able to understand and speak either English, Zulu, Xhosa or Setswana as those were the languages in which the interviewer was able to communicate.

Convenience purposive sampling (Abdellah & Levine, 1979) was used. Mediators asked for volunteers in the township who complied with the criteria of the sample to participate in the research. The first two volunteers were selected from each of the five sections of the township. The size of the sample was 10 individuals.

The phenomenological method (Burns & Grove, 1987) of interviewing was used to gather data. The researcher conducted an unstructured interview asking one question to each individual being interviewed: 'What is your experience of exposure to violence, especially the violence that has taken place since March 1990?' Each interview was audiotaped and lasted about 45 minutes. Communication techniques like probing, paraphrasing, summarizing, reflecting, minimal responding and clarifying were used to encourage individuals to ventilate freely. Field notes were made immediately after each interview to describe the whole situation of the interview and the researcher's impressions.

## Pilot study

A pilot study was conducted by interviewing two individuals who met the criteria of the study. This was done to identify any possible stumbling blocks that would be encountered in this type of research. Thereafter, the rest of the interviews were conducted. The tape recordings of the interviews were transcribed verbatim and the data were analysed using Kerlinger's (1986) method of content analysis. The researcher first read through all the transcriptions and identified the universal categories of the data and defined them. Next, units of analysis were identified from the data by underlining words and themes that were placed in the identified universal categories. Words and themes were then categorized.

The transcriptions of the tape recordings were then given to another psychiatric nursing specialist with a protocol on how to analyse the data. The researcher and psychiatric nursing specialist then met to compare their analyses and agree on categories of units of analysis. The categories were then prioritized, based on how many individuals experienced the same aspects.

## Results

The universum of the study was all the verbal responses of the respondents. The universum was then categorized as follows:

(1) Psychological experiences. All the observations, investigations and recordings of the mind and its function are defined as psychological experiences. The mind is the organized total of psychological processes and contents that allow the individual to respond to external and internal stimuli in an integrated and dynamic way relating response to the present to both the past and the future of the individual. The processes of perceiving, learning, thinking, feeling and behaving with intelligence are its principal processes. The contents of the mind vary with experience (*Chambers*, 1974; *Churchill*, 1989; Madela, 1991).

(2) Spiritual experience. This is the moral and religious influences on behaviour as reflected in values, ethical principles and relationships within the community (*Longman*, 1984).

(3) Physical experiences. Physical experiences are those that pertain to the body. They also relate to structure, size or shape of something that can be touched and seen (*Collins*, 1984).

(4) Behavioural experiences. Behavioural experiences pertain to the entire complex of observable, recordable and measurable activities of an individual as a result of his/her relationships with various features of his/her environment; in other words, anything the individual does (*Chambers*, 1974, Madela, 1991, Stuart & Sudeen, 1991).

### Coding

Coding was done by underlining all words and themes that were used in the transcriptions, classifying them into universal categories and clustering them into subcategories. A protocol was then drawn up and given to a psychiatric nursing specialist who also did coding independently, following the same steps. Afterwards, the researcher and the psychiatric nurse specialist met and discussed the results until a consensus was reached regarding categorization.

The results indicated that the respondents had negative and positive experiences (Madela, 1991) (see Table 6.1). According to the researcher's

**Table 6.1** The experience of a community characterized by violence (Madela 1991).

| Negative experiences | | Positive experiences |
| --- | --- | --- |
| *1. Patterns of interaction within internal environment* | | |
| Perceptions of: | confusion | |
| | uselessness | |
| | dehumanization | |
| | inability to forget | |
| | repression | |
| | sad feelings | |
| | empty feelings | |
| | fear | |
| Spiritual | disorganization: of family lives, education, productivity and interpersonal relationships. | Improvement: in employer–employee relationship and in faith |
| | Lack: of basic needs and trust | |
| Physical loss: | of lives, sleep, accommodation, property and jobs. | |
| | Deterioration: in services and physical health. | |
| *2. Patterns of interaction between internal and external environment* | | |
| Intrapersonal | Pretence | Increased appreciation, Bravery |
| Interpersonal | Thuggery | Solidarity |
| | Scapegoating | |
| | Harassment | |

definition of a community, the experiences represent both internal and external environments. The internal environment, according to the researcher's metatheoretical assumption, consists of all the psychological, spiritual and physical aspects of the community; the external environment consists of the behaviour that results from the interactions between the internal environment and external environment. The individual's health affects the health of the community and the community reflects the individual's health.

Data showed many negative experiences in the internal environment with only two positive experiences, i.e. improvements in employer–employee relationships and in faith, which are spiritual experiences. All the psychological experiences, most of the spiritual experiences and all the physical experiences expressed were negative. Thus, overall, the respondents' internal environments were negatively affected. In the external environment, especially in intrapersonal behaviour, more positive than negative experiences were expressed. Although the situation was perceived as threatening and overwhelming, the positive experiences of increased appreciation and bravery were remarkable: 'I was lucky to be alive'. The situation opened the people's minds to the fact that it was an advantage for them to have each other, and thus they started appreciating each other more than before: 'My mother was just holding her breath when I was out fighting, praying that I should come back alive, and I also kept on going back home to check if they were still alive'.

**Bravery**

Bravery, another positive behaviour within self, was felt by most who appreciated the seriousness of the situation and gained courage to bring about change. In interpersonal behaviour, though, there were many negative experiences that resulted from the interaction in the negative internal environments: 'They would loot people's properties in broad daylight'. The only positive interpersonal behaviour was that of solidarity, which shows that those 'terrifying' conditions, as one respondent put it, made people find common ground, and therefore stand by one another.

In analysing the field notes made by the field worker it seemed that, generally, all the respondents were open and seemingly honest with the researcher. It was remarkable, though, that all the respondents were initially suspicious and unyielding because of the impact of violence on their lives. This suspicion was overcome by the fact that most of the respondents knew the researcher's relatives well and so gained insight with explanation. Those who knew the researcher as well, five of the 10, were more than willing to help, but had to obtain strong reassurance by asking many questions to be able to share each 'sensitive' information, as one put it.

Five respondents, those who did not know the researcher, still sounded suspicious even after they had consented; they still held the intermediaries responsible for any trouble they would get into as a result of the inter-views. All the respondents seemed emotional when they talked of their experiences and seemed to relive them; some even became tearful. This was also evident in the type of language they used, impolite as it would be in the real situation.

Another remarkable aspect was the difference between the time it took to obtain co-operation from the older respondents in contrast to younger respondents. The older respondents still appeared very suspicious until the intermediaries of their age explained once more, to help them to feel secure. Eight respondents seemed to regard 'violence' as the political–tribal war that hit the township at the time specified in the comprehensive question, although nine of the respondents agreed that they still did not feel totally safe at the time of the interview, more than a year after the onset of that violence (Madela, 1991).

## Discussion

The results of this study indicated that the experience of violence by the victims could be psychological, spiritual, physical and behavioural. This fact agrees with Lazarus' statement, as used by Van den Bos & Bryant (1987) in their study of human response to disasters, in which he wrote of a field of stress, encompassing physiological, sociological and psychological phenomena. Madela (1991) differs in discussing the results of this study, by categorizing similar human responses that Van den Bos & Bryant (1987) have placed under social responses, under spiritual responses. From an African viewpoint unhealthy stress responses always incorporate elements of disharmony with the human spirit, with the family and with village society (Atkins, 1984).

### Correlation with other findings

The experiences of victims correlated exactly with the results of a study conducted by Loughrey *et al.* (1988) on victims of civil violence in Northern Ireland, the results of a study conducted by Gibson (1986) on the effects of civil unrest on children, the factors identified as reactions of victims of violence by Haegert (1990) and those identified by Organization for Appropriate Social Services in South Africa (OASSSA) (n.d.) as responses to stress after having studied the forces that cause stress in a township continually. The results of all these studies led to the identification of post-traumatic stress disorder in each case. The recent research by Simpson (1992) and Eagle (1992) supports the findings that victims of violence are likely to develop post-traumatic stress disorder.

The results of this study also correlate with the facts given by Vogelman (1990), in a study conducted on workers, from which he identified the effects of violence on the individuals living in a community saturated by violence. Grange (1990) quoted Vogelman's statement on the tragedy of Natal that police were not seen to be exercising law and order.

This was one of the findings of the study under discussion in the township of interest. One respondent stated, 'I will never trust the police again'. Anon. (1990b) also quoted a young person from the squatter settlement indicated in this study reflecting distrust of the police, saying 'They [police] are going to take our weapons to the hostels and give them to Zulus'.

Singh (1990) wrote of a survey conducted by Duke in the Pretoria, Witwatersrand and Vaaltriangle townships. He took a sample of workers which revealed that, apart from the extremely high levels of stress owing to the unrest, other factors such as inadequate housing, the education crisis, evictions, fear of violence and theft, and lack of sleep are factors contributing to stress levels. These factors were also revealed by the present study, and they put the community at risk and correlate with emotional disorder according to Murray & Huelskoeter (1987).

Ndabandaba (1988) conducted a study on crimes of violence in the Umlazi township, and, although he concentrated on the physical effects of violence in detail, the study under discussion revealed some of these in the physical experience category of its results. It was striking to note that this study revealed all the impacts of violence on the victims, as discussed by McKendrick & Hoffman (1990) after comparing the results of research of other people done on victims of violence both within South Africa and outside. The results of this study and their comparison to other researchers' results lead to a diagnosis of post-traumatic stress disorder for the community studied, as tabulated by the American Psychiatric Association (in Kaplan & Sadock, 1989). The results of this study matched all the different categories of the diagnostic criteria for post-traumatic stress disorder.

The results correlate with the description in category A in that the respondents experienced an event that was outside the range of usual human experience and that proved to be markedly distressing to almost anyone. The experiences revealed were, for example, serious threat to one's life or physical integrity, serious threat or harm to one's children, spouse, home and community, seeing another person who had recently been, or was killed or seriously injured, and many others that had the same effects as these.

The description in category B pertaining to the persistent re-experiencing of the traumatic event corresponds with the results indicating recurrent and intrusive distressing recollections of the event by most people, suddenly acting or feeling as if the traumatic events were recurring.

The results can be compared to the description in category C in that they revealed persistent avoidance of stimuli associated with the trauma (as one respondent stated, 'I no longer take taxis that go via the hostels') and numbing of general responses, as indicated by efforts to avoid thoughts and feelings associated with the trauma, efforts to avoid activities and situations that arouse recollections of the trauma, feeling of detachment and estrangement from others, and a sense of a foreshortened future.

The results correspond to the description in category D in that they showed persistent symptoms of increased arousal which were not present before the trauma: difficulty in falling asleep, hypervigilance and physiological reactivity. For example, they expressed an experience of running for cover when hearing people screaming outside.

The results compare to category E in that the disturbances lasted far more than one month. The results also revealed that the behaviour of the victims of violence was a result of the interaction of the physical, spiritual and psychological experiences which make the internal environment.

These three aspects were advocated by Lazarus (in Van den Bos & Bryant, 1987) as components of a field of stress which then, according to these two authors, impacts on behaviour. The results also indicated that stress is neither a stimulus nor a response (Lazarus, in Van den Bos & Bryant, 1987) in that respondents revealed an experience of stress both when they were victims and when they were victimizers. This was revealed in one respondent's words regarding both situations: 'I was jumping fences with fear, just running so that they could not find me'. At the time he went with a group of people to kill people at the hostel, 'I was literally frozen, it was unsafe inside and unsafe outside, so the best thing was to go inside and kill my enemies'.

## Positive effects

It was interesting to note from the results of this study that, although a number of researchers had proven that violence has negative effects on the victims (Gibson, 1986; Haegert, 1990; Loughrey *et al.*, 1988; OASSSA n.d.), it does also have positive effects. This was revealed by respondents who expressed an experience of solidarity which had resulted from the feeling of being 'one' in suffering and therefore strengthening one another to stand the suffering.

Bravery as a behaviour was also revealed in the study by respondents who noticed how helpless other victims were in the situation and became determined to do whatever was in their power to save the situation. The violent situation also brought out a behaviour of increased appreciation in the victims in that, in the midst of these helplessly overwhelming conditions, they learnt to appreciate what they had when compared with others: the fact that they were still alive after so many people had died, the fact that their families were still with them and not wandering out somewhere looking for places to hide, and that they were not some of the more sought-after people.

From the results of this study, it appears that the internal environment of the victims of violence is generally negative (Madela, 1991). Taking into consideration the three components of the internal environment, i.e. the psychological, the spiritual and the physical environment, it follows that the only positive experiences in the whole internal environment were the improvement in employer–employee relationships ($n = 6$) and in faith ($n = 6$).

The results of the study also showed that the external environment, i.e. behaviour, which results from interactions between the internal environment and external environment consisted of both positive and negative experiences (Madela, 1991). This means that, even though the internal environment was predominantly negative and hopeless, the victims still had that subconscious will to survive in the situation. This showed in their positive behaviour, which was their only hope and means of survival.

Figure 6.1 illustrates how interactions among the components of the internal environment and external environment affected the respondents' behaviour. In the case of the victims of violence, the psychological, spiritual

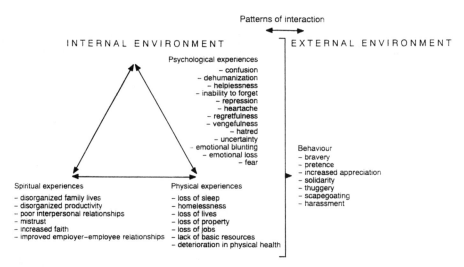

Patterns of interaction

INTERNAL ENVIRONMENT        EXTERNAL ENVIRONMENT

Psychological experiences
  – confusion
  – dehumanization
  – helplessness
  – inability to forget
  – repression
  – heartache
  – regretfulness
  – vengefulness
  – hatred
  – uncertainty
  – emotional blunting
  – emotional loss
  – fear

Behaviour
  – bravery
  – pretence
  – increased appreciation
  – solidarity
  – thuggery
  – scapegoating
  – harassment

Spiritual experiences
  – disorganized family lives
  – disorganized productivity
  – poor interpersonal relationships
  – mistrust
  – increased faith
  – improved employer–employee relationships

Physical experiences
  – loss of sleep
  – homelessness
  – loss of lives
  – loss of property
  – loss of jobs
  – lack of basic resources
  – deterioration in physical health

**Fig. 6.1**   Patterns of interaction in the environment of a community exposed to violence (Madela 1991).

and physical experiences interacted with the external environment and then resulted in behaviour which is then shown to the outside, either in the victim's conduct or in his interactions with people around him.

The overall experience of the respondents in this study leads to the conclusion that the whole community, after being exposed to violence, was already suffering from post-traumatic stress disorder, because the individual experiences expressed match all the categories listed in the diagnostic criteria for post-traumatic stress disorder (Madela, 1991).

The community exposed to violence was continuously experiencing stress. Stress in this study was experienced by the community in two contexts: as a stimulus for violence and as a response to violence. It then followed that stress goes hand-in-hand with violence, but it was neither a stimulus nor a response, since the victims showed signs and symptoms of stress both before and after exposure to violence.

## Practical problems

Practical problems encountered during this research include unwillingness of some subjects to participate in the research and problems with public communication resources. Because of the sensitivity of the topic of research, some subjects made many excuses not to be interviewed, either because they did not want to recall the most fearsome situation in their lives, or because they were suspicious that the information they divulged might get them into trouble with the police.

When data collection was started, the township was still in darkness and the telephones were not working, which delayed the process of data gathering because the means of communication became poor. Some subjects agreed to be interviewed, but it was difficult for them to inform the researcher of changes that required postponements of the interview. Others would return late from work when it was unsafe for the researcher to reach them.

## Recommendations

Recommendations are made based on the findings of this study by referring to the applicability of the study in terms of nursing education, nursing practice and nursing research.

Although this study had some limitations, caused by practical problems encountered, it also had possibilities of application for the future. The results of this study deserve to be included in the curriculum for psychiatric nursing, particularly in community psychiatric nursing, both at undergraduate and postgraduate levels. These results can also be included in the curriculum for community health nursing, as the community nurse is concerned with the well-being of the community at all levels. The multi-disciplinary team can also benefit from the findings of this study when dealing with victims of violence when they have already developed mental illness and have been admitted to the psychiatric wards.

## A challenge for psychiatric nurses

In practice, these findings should challenge psychiatric nurses to put more emphasis on support action that focuses on the promotion of mental health and prevention of mental illness in the community; that is to use their body of knowledge, both theoretical and practical, to plan and carry out programmes for prevention of violence through community development, and providing treatment for post-traumatic stress disorder.

### Prevention of violence through community development

This can be done by creating opportunities for ordinary people of all ages to explore and transform those facets of their own lives and environments that may have been distorted by the experience of apartheid and violence (Seedat *et al.*, 1992). These facets include reconstruction of education, employment creation, anti-crime and anti-gang initiatives, reforming the prison system, psychological healing, and rebuilding of authority structures that are acceptable to all (Mokwena, 1992; Ramphele, 1992).

**Providing treatment for post-traumatic stress disorder**

Early treatment within the context of a supportive community can provide effective and lasting relief. The psychiatric nurse's monitoring of the careful use of appropriate psychotropic drugs can be invaluable in providing effective therapy. This will enable survivors of violence to fully participate and benefit from individual psychotherapy (Simpson, 1992).

*Psychotherapy*

Short term individual psychotherapy, consisting of two to three sessions, assists the survivor of violence to ventilate feelings and regain a sense of self-sufficiency. The psychiatric nurse solicits information, offers support and affirmation and serves in an educative function (Eagle, 1992; Dlamini, 1992).

*Group therapy*

Group therapy is also a valuable resource in treating post-traumatic stress disorder. Moloto (1993), a psychiatric nurse, conducted eight sessions of group nursing therapy with six female adolescents exposed to violence who presented with depression and failure to progress at school. Initially the adolescents voiced despair and perceived themselves as helpless victims of violence. As the group therapy progressed the adolescents perceived themselves as becoming more in charge of their lives and were able to manage constructively stress caused by violence.

*Theatre*

Popular theatre can also be used, where the traumatized act out their own experiences. The psychiatric nurse can also educate the community about the dynamics of violence and how survivors of violence can be reintegrated in the community (Dlamini, 1992).

**Further research**

To date, the literature is limited and very little research has been done on the subject of a community's experience of violence. The possibilities of applying the results of this study in nursing research are unlimited, and it has actually opened doors to further research. This study has left unanswered questions like the experience of the police and of the hostel dwellers, of the violence, since in the study these two groups were pointed out as perpetrators of all the trouble.

The effects of the violence on children is another area which needs attention, since they were the most helpless victims of the whole situation, and they have different experiences from the adult population. The other question that still needs to be answered is the role of the municipal council in the violence in the township, because the results of this study indicated a lot of passivity in, if not neglect of, their role in the services they normally render.

In conclusion, the findings of this research study can successfully be utilized in nursing education and practice and also for follow-up research projects.

## *References*

Abdellah, F. & Levine, E. (1979) *Better Patient Care Through Nursing Research*, 2nd edn, p. 333. McMillan, New York.

Anders, T. & Hlophe, S. (1990) Violence in Black townships. *The Star*, 30 August, p. 1, C1–C3.

Anon. (1990a) Leaders' first task; help halt violence. *The Star*, 14 March, p. 16, C1–C2.

Anon. (1990b) Disarmed and trapped. *The Star*, 16 August, p. 17, C1–C5.

Atkins, T. (1984) What is health? *Health and Development*, Summer, 4–7.

Burgers, L. (1990) Health must be ensured. *The Star*, 30 August, p. 1, C3–C4.

Burns, N. & Grove, S. (1987) *The Practice of Nursing Research: Conduct, Critique and Utilisation*, pp. 39–40. W.B. Saunders, Philadelphia.

*Chambers 20th Century Dictionary* (1974), pp. 116, 949. Chambers, Cambridge.

*Churchill's Medical Dictionary* (1989), p. 1168. Churchill Livingstone, New York.

*Collins English Language Dictionary* (1984), p. 1077. Collins, London.

Dlamini, B. (1992) The Imbali rehabilitation programme. *Critical Health*, **41**, 56–8

Eagle, G. (1992) Violence and mental health: post-traumatic stress and depression. *Critical Health*, **41**, 41–6.

Gibson, K. (1986) *The Effects of Civil Unrest on Children*, pp. 14–111. Cape Town University Press, Cape Town.

Grange, H. (1990) Where violence conflict has become way of life. *The Star*, 16 August, p. 10, C2–C5.

Haegert, S. (1990) The victims of violence. *Nursing RSA*, **5**(8), 18–21.

Kaplan, H.I. & Sadock, B.J. (1989) *Comprehensive Textbook of Psychiatry*, 5th edn., pp. 1000–1001. Williams and Wilkins, Baltimore.

Kerlinger, F. (1986) *Foundations of Behavioral Research*, pp. 477–83. Holt, Reinhart and Winston, New York.

Lab, S. (1988) *The Psychological Effects of Unrest Conditions on Children, With Specific Reference to S.A. Townships*, p. 16. University of the Witwatersrand, Johannesburg.

*Longman Dictionary of Psychology and Psychiatry* (1984), p. 705. Longman, New York.

Loughrey, G.C., Bell, P., Kee, M., Roddy, R.G. & Curran, P.S. (1988) Post-traumatic stress disorder and civil violence in Northern Ireland. *British Journal of Psychiatry*, **153**, 554–60.

McKendrick, B. & Hoffman, W. (1990) *People and Violence in South Africa*, pp. 27–29. Oxford University Press, Cape Town.

Madela, E.N. (1991) Guideline for supportive action by a psychiatric nurse in a community exposed to violence. Unpublished mini-dissertation MCur (Psychiatric Nursing), Rand Afrikaans University, Johannesburg, pp. 1–77.

Mokwena, S. (1992) Living on the wrong side of the law: marginalisation, youth and violence. In *Black Youth in Crisis: Facing the future* (eds D. Everatt & E. Sisulu), pp. 45–49. Ravan, Braamfontein.

Moloto, J.C. (1993) Facilitating the mental health of adolescents exposed to violence by group nursing therapy. Unpublished mini-dissertation for credit towards MCur. (Psychiatric Nursing), pp. 1–90. Rand Afrikaans University, Johannesburg.

Mouton, J. & Marais, H. (1989) *Basic Concepts in the Methodology of the Social Sciences*, pp. 43–9. Human Sciences Research Council, Pretoria.

Murray, R. & Huelskoeter, M. (1987) *Psychiatric–Mental Health Nursing*, 2nd edn, pp. 619–79. Prentice Hall, Englewood Cliffs, New Jersey.

Ndabandaba, G.L. (1988) *Crimes of Violence in Black Townships*, p. 72. Butterworths, Durban.

OASSSA (n.d.) *Repression and Stress: a Handbook*, pp. 3–7. OASSSA, Johannesburg.

Poggenpoel, M. (1984) *Die Funksies van die Psigiatriese Verpleegkundige in Suid-Afrika*, p. 44. Juta, Cape Town.

Ramphele, M. (1992) Social disintegration in the black community: implications of social transformation. In *Black Youth in Crisis: Facing the future* (eds D. Everatt & E. Sisulu), pp. 10–28. Ravan, Braamfontein.

Seedat, M., Terre Blanche, M., Butchart, A., & Dell, V. (1992) Violence prevention through community development: the centre for peace action model. *Critical Health*, **41**, 59–64.

Simpson, M. (1992) Post-traumatic stress disorder: a response to abnormal circumstances. *Critical Health*, **41**, 36–40.

Singh, S. (1990) Townships' stress inhibits productivity. *The Star*, 23 August, p. 14, C1–C4.

Smith, C. (1990) Violence in a sick society. *New Nation*, 8 March, p. 23, C1–C6.

Stuart, G.W. & Sudeen, S.J. (1987) *Principles and Practice of Psychiatric Nursing*, 3rd edn., p. 37. C.V. Mosby, St Louis.

Stuart, G.W. & Sudeen, S.J. (1991) *Principles and Practice of Psychiatric Nursing*, 4th edn., p. 1005. C.V. Mosby, St Louis.

Van den Bos, V. & Bryant, B. (1987) *Cataclysm, Crises and Catastrophes. Psychology in Action*, p. 65. American Psychological Association, Washington.

Vogelman, L. (1986) An opening speech, 3. OASSSA National Conference, Johannesburg, 17–18 May.

Vogelman, L. (1990) Workers affected by violence need business' aid, *Business Day*, 9 November, p. 1, Col. 1–5.

Woods, N.F. & Catanzaro, M. (1988) *Nursing Research: Theory and Practice*, pp. 136–137. C.V. Mosby, St. Louis.

# Chapter 7
# The care and handling of peripheral intravenous cannulae on 60 surgery and internal medicine patients: an observation study

ANNA LUNDGREN, *RN, BA*

Lecturer, College of the Health Professions, Department of Caring Sciences

LENNART JORFELDT, *MD, PhD*

Professor, Health Care Research, Department of Clinical Physiology

and ANNA-CHRISTINA EK, *RN, BSc, DMSc*

Associate Professor, Department of Caring Sciences, Faculty of Health Sciences, Linköping University, Linköping, Sweden

The purpose of this study was to analyse the actual routines surrounding the use of peripheral IV cannulae and the occurrence of complications. Thirty surgery patients and 30 internal medicine patients were observed daily at a medium-sized hospital. The patients were followed from the time the cannula was inserted until after withdrawal and until both the insertion site and the vein were free from pain. The results showed that most of the cannulae were placed on the upper side of the hand and sizes most frequently used were 1.0 and 1.2 mm. The fixation was already unsatisfactory in 23 cases after the second day. Twenty-three cannulae were removed after 24 hours. Thirty-seven patients (62%) were stated to have thrombophlebitis in different degrees. Only seven cannulae fulfilled the criteria for good cannula care and handling. The frequency of complication was especially high when fructose–glucose, antibiotics or anticoagulants were given. There was no documentation in the patient record, contrary to current laws in Sweden. The complications observed were redness, swelling, haematoma, subcutaneous swelling and suppurating infection. The study showed that the longer the cannula had been *in situ*, the greater were the complications (very distinct after 24 hours). The care and handling was unsatisfactory to very unsatisfactory in 52% of the cases. Complications can last for a very long time. In this research, pain was noted up to five months after the cannulae were removed.

## *Introduction*

A disposable membrane cannula was introduced in 1963 and at the time was mainly used for intensive care (Mossberg, 1981). Today, the insertion and care of peripheral cannulae is a routine task for nurses in all kinds of care. Intravenous IV routines are considered for administration of nutrition, infusion solutions, cytotoxic drugs, blood, etc. (MacFarlane *et al.*, 1980; Maki & Band, 1981).

Several studies have reported complications related to the use of peripheral cannulae (Hästbacka *et al.*, 1966; Maki & Martin, 1975; Hessov *et al.*, 1977; Hessov, 1985; Wildsmith, 1978; Buxton *et al.*, 1979; Smallman *et al.*, 1980; MacFarlane *et al.*, 1980, 1981; Hedstrand & Zaren, 1989; Nordenström *et al.*, 1991). The complications which have been reported are local tenderness, signs of inflammation, thrombophlebitis and infection (Brismar & Nyström, 1986; Maki *et al.*, 1978; Mossberg, 1988) presumably caused mainly by chemical, but also by bacteriological, effects in the vessels (Hamory, 1987).

### Thrombophlebitis

Most interest has been paid to thrombophlebitis, about which there are different opinions as to development and appearance. The scale of symptoms given for thrombophlebitis (Th) varies among the different authors but includes tenderness, redness, pain, swelling, increased temperature, hard vein, increasing pain, spreading redness and possibly fever (Brismar & Nyström, 1986; von Dardel *et al.*, 1986). Bergqvist (1971) defined thrombophlebitis on a scale of four, ranging from slight discomfort and light tenderness to palpable thrombus, erythema, burning and continuous prolonged discomfort, whilst Maddox & Rush (1977) proposed a five-grade scale to be able to grade the degree of severity of thrombophlebitis.

Thrombophlebitis is supposed to develop within 12 to 24 hours, but mostly does not appear until after two to six days (von Dardel *et al.*, 1986, Mossberg, 1986, 1988). According to Maddox & Rush (1977), thrombophlebitis can be defined and classified in different degrees.

Different studies show different figures regarding the frequency of thrombophlebitis. The incidence of thrombophlebitis increases as the number of hours the cannula is *in situ* increases (Maki *et al.*, 1978, von Dardel *et al.*, 1986). Only a few cases were registered when the cannulae were *in situ* for less than 12 hours, while the frequency was 70% when the cannulae were *in situ* for more than 72 hours (Collins *et al.*, 1975). With infusion times exceeding 96 hours, almost all patients developed thrombophlebitis (Nordenström *et al.*, 1991). No studies have reported the duration of the thrombophlebitis or symptoms related to the complications.

Additional factors pointed out as needing attention in the prevention of complications are the location and size of the cannulae, hygiene, their fixation and the infusion of vein irritants (Spanos, 1976; Hecher *et al.*, 1976; Hecher, 1980; Lodge *et al.*, 1987; Mossberg, 1986, 1988). The most common locations reported earlier are on the upper side of the hand or forehand and the recommended size should be small enough to permit blood to flow around the catheter (MacFarlane *et al.*, 1980; Maki & Band, 1981). For the daily administration of one to three litres of fluid, a size of 0.8 mm is recommended as being quite sufficient (Hecher *et al.*, 1976; Spanos, 1976; Spanos & Hecher, 1979; von Dardel *et al.*, 1986; Mossberg, 1986, 1988). Hypo- and hypertonic solutions and blood are considered as vein irritants.

When a cannula is inserted, it has to be cared for daily by the nurses. Signs which reflect the degree of care are hygiene and fixation and dressing of the cannula and the time it has been *in situ* (MacFarlane *et al.*, 1980, 1981; Smallman *et al.*, 1980). Studies reflecting the relation between the development of complications and the actual care and handling of the cannulae are rare.

## The study

The purpose of the study was to describe the frequency of thrombophlebitis in surgery and internal medicine wards related to IV cannulae location, size, time *in situ* and the care and handling of peripheral cannulae. The purpose was also to study the duration of the symptoms.

### Subjects

The study was carried out in a medium-sized hospital and included 60 patients, 30 from each of surgery and internal medicine wards. The inclusion criteria were that a cannula had been inserted into the patient the day the observations should start and that the patient was able to understand and answer the questions adequately. The only exclusion criterion was that the patients received temporary care exceeding 20 hours on some other ward.

### Procedure

The patient's sex, age, diagnosis and drugs were registered along with the days of insertion and removal of the cannula, its size, location, fixation and dressing. The patients were diagnosed by the physicians according to the International Classification of Diseases system (ICD-9) (1986). Drugs and solutions were classified into groups according to *Pharmaceutical Specialities in Sweden* (1991).

During the time the peripheral cannula was *in situ* in the vein, the care and handling, infused fluids, complications and symptoms indicated by the patients were observed. When a complication was registered, observation of the patient's symptoms continued even after removal of the cannula, until the patient was reported free of the symptoms. If the patient's complications remained on discharge, contact continued by means of regular telephone interviews, at the longest for up to six months. Even the patient's own experience of the peripheral cannula was registered.

One observer has performed all the observations and made assessments according to given criteria concerning the ranking and the care and handling.

## Definitions

Thrombophlebitis in this study was defined as follows:

Degree 0    *No complications*
            None or slight discomfort;
            tenderness at insertion
Degree 1    *Light thrombophlebitis*
            Red area and tenderness
Degree 2    *Medium thrombophlebitis*
            Red area, tenderness, pain and slight swelling
Degree 3    *Severe thrombophlebitis*
            Red area, tenderness, pain, swelling more than 2 × 4 cm;
            increased temperature in the area and palpable chord in the vein
Degree 4    *Very severe thrombophlebitis*
            Red area, pain, swelling more than 5 × 8 cm;
            increased temperature in the area;
            palpable chord in the vein;
            pain spreading up to the arm, red string and, possibly, fever.

The nurse's care and handling of peripheral cannulae were defined as follows:

Degree 0    *Satisfactory care and handling*
            Good fixation and clean;
            patient without pain
Degree 1    *Less satisfactory care and handling*
            Fixed cannula with loose wings or i.v. line;
            incomplete dressing;
            the cannula moves visibly in the vein when the patient moves his arm;
            the patient mentions that the cannula is touching the inside of the vein;
            blood on the outside of cannula plug and/or dressing
Degree 2    *Unsatisfactory care and handling*

The cannula is unsatisfactorily fixed or not fixed at all;
incomplete dressing;
the cannula can move in the vein and the patient mentions that
the cannula is touching the vein and at the place of insertion;
blood on the outside of cannula plug and/or dressing

Degree 3    *Very unsatisfactory care and handling*
Non-functioning fixation of the cannula;
only the dressing holds the cannula in place;
the cannula can move in the vein and the patient mentions that
the cannula is touching the vein and at the place of insertion;
the cannula is *in situ* more than 5 days.

## Type of peripheral intravenous cannula (PIV)

Type of I.V. cannula used was Venflon I.V. cannula, from BOC OHMEDA, Helsingborg, Sweden.

## Statistical methods

The data are presented as the mean $\pm$ SD or the median (Md). Students' *t*-test, the Chi-square test and Fischer's exact test have been applied.

## *Results*

Thirty-eight patients were male, 22 female and their age was $61.0 \pm 16.9$ years, range 21 to 91. The patients in the surgery wards were older, $66.0 \pm 14.6$, than the patients in the internal medicine wards, $56.0 \pm 18.7$ ($P < 0.02$) (Table 7.1). The diagnoses are presented in Table 7.2.

The most frequently used cannula sizes were 1.0 mm (20 gauge) $n = 37$ (60%) and 1.2 mm (18 gauge) $n = 17$ (28%). Three of the cannulae were 0.8

**Table 7.1**   The incidence of thrombophlebitis (Th) in relation to age and sex for 60 patients from surgery and internal medicine wards.

| Age | Surgery | Th | Male | Female | Internal medicine | Th | Male | Female |
|---|---|---|---|---|---|---|---|---|
| 20–39 | 1 | — | — | — | 11 | 8 | 2 | 6 |
| 40–59 | 7 | 4 | 4 | | 2 | 2 | 2 | — |
| 60–79 | 17 | 10 | 6 | 4 | 15 | 10 | 10 | — |
| 80–99 | 5 | 2 | 2 | — | 2 | 1 | — | 1 |
| Total | $n = 30$ | 16 | 12 | 4 | $n = 30$ | 21 | 14 | 7 |

**Table 7.2**  Diagnosis of the 60 patients observed on the surgery and internal medicine wards.

| Sugery | | Internal medicine | |
|---|---|---|---|
| Sinusitis | 1 | Asthma | 2 |
| Hernia | 1 | Angina | 2 |
| Abdominal obs. | 2 | Haematemesis | 2 |
| By-pass op. | 3 | Colon X-ray | 1 |
| Causa socialis | 1 | Cerebral vascular disease | 1 |
| Gastroscopy | 1 | Diabetes | 3 |
| Haemorrhoids | 1 | Borelia | 1 |
| Hip joint op. | 3 | Heart infarction | 7 |
| Icterus | 2 | Muscle rupture, leg | 3 |
| Ileus | 3 | Crohn's disease | 1 |
| Neo mammae | 1 | Thrombosis in the neck | 2 |
| Pancreatitis | 2 | Thrombosis in the leg | 1 |
| Pancreas cancer | 2 | Ulcerous colitis | 1 |
| Prostrate | 1 | Skin rash, foot | 3 |
| Intestinal bleeding | 1 | | |
| Transural resection | 2 | | |
| Urinary tract stone | 1 | | |
| Left leg op. | 1 | | |
| Ear op. | 1 | | |
| Total | $n = 30$ | | $n = 30$ |

(22 gauge) and three were larger than 1.2 mm. The number of larger cannulae used was significantly higher in the surgery wards ($P < 0.02$) (Table 7.3).

The majority of the cannulae, 40 (67%), were placed on the upper side of the hand and the most common method of fixation was a sterile non-occlusive dressing, commonly in combination with a gauze dressing, $n = 39$ (65%). Of the 37 cannulae which remained *in situ* more than 24 hours, the fixation was unsatisfactory on the second day on 17 (46%) of the patients and, of the 22 (37%) which remained *in situ* more than 48 hours, 12 (55%) were unsatisfactorily fixed or not fixed at all the third day. Of 10 cannulae which remained *in situ* for 72 hours (three days and nights) or more, six (60%) were unsatisfactorily fixed or not fixed at all the fourth day, and of the six which remained *in situ* 96 hours (four days and nights) or more, five (83%) were unsatisfactorily or very unsatisfactorily fixed the fifth day.

## Complications

Of 40 cannulae placed on the upper side of the hand, 15 (37%) were 1.2 mm or larger. Nine of these caused complications: three light thrombophlebitis (degree 1), two severe thrombophlebitis (degree 3) and two very severe thrombophlebitis (degree 4). There was no significant difference in the thrombophlebitis frequency between the wards and sexes.

Twenty-three cannulae (38%) were removed after 24 hours, 15 (25%) after

**Table 7.3**  Number of cannulae in relation to size and thrombophlebitis (Th) for 60 patients in surgery and internal medicine wards.

| Size/gauge | Number | Surgery | Internal medicine | Degree of thrombophlebitis | | | | | Th % |
| | | | | 0 | 1 | 2 | 3 | 4 | |
|---|---|---|---|---|---|---|---|---|---|
| 0.8/22 | 3 (5%) | — | 3 | — | 2 | — | 1 | — | 8 |
| 1.0/20 | 37 (62%) | 15 | 22 | 14 | 9 | 5 | 7 | 2 | 62 |
| 1.2/18 | 17 (28%) | 13 | 4 | 9 | 2 | 3 | 1 | 2 | 22 |
| 1.4/17 | 1 (2%) | 1 | — | — | — | 1 | — | — | 3 |
| 1.7/16 | 1 (2%) | 1 | — | — | — | 1 | — | — | 3 |
| 2.0/14 | 1 (2%) | — | 1 | — | — | — | 1 | — | 3 |
| Total | $n = 60$ | 30 | 30 | 23 | 13 | 10 | 10 | 4 | |

48 hours, and 22 (37%) after 72–168 hours (3–7 days) (Fig. 7.1). In the internal medicine wards, the patients' cannulae were *in situ* in the vein significantly longer (Md = 3 days) than in the surgery ward (Md = 1 day) ($P < 0.01$).

Thirty-seven (62%) cannulae caused thrombophlebitis of different degrees. For the patients with the cannula *in situ* for up to 24 hours, $n = 23$ (37%), the frequency of thrombophlebitis was significantly lower than for the other patients. Of these 23, 11 (47%) had thrombophlebitis ($P < 0.01$). Of 37 patients who had the cannula *in situ* for 48 hours or longer, 29 (78%) had thrombophlebitis, of which nine (31%) were considered severe or very severe. Seventeen (77%) of 22 (37%) patients who had the cannula *in situ* for

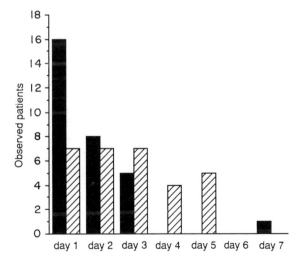

**Fig. 7.1**  The number of days the peripheral cannulae have been *in situ* on 60 observed patients on surgery (■) and internal medicine (▨) wards.

**Table 7.4**  Development of thrombophlebitis (Th) in relation to drugs given and infusion for 60 patients at surgery and internal medicine wards.

|  | Number of patients | Number of patients with Th |
|---|---|---|
| Drugs |  |  |
| Antibiotics | 12 | 9 |
| Anticoagulants | 5 | 5 |
| Solutions |  |  |
| Glucose | 11 | 10 |
| Fructose–glucose | 4 | 2 |
| Rehydrex | 15 | 5 |
| Blood | 3 | 1 |
| Remainder | 9 | 4 |
| No drugs | 1 | 1 |
| Total | $n = 60$ | 37 |

72 hours or more had thrombophlebitis of different degrees. Of 10 (60%) which had the cannula *in situ* for 96 hours (four days and nights) or more, nine (90%) had thrombophlebitis and six (10%) of those with the cannula *in situ* for 120 hours (five days and nights) or more all manifested thrombophlebitis, according to the definition given.

The frequency of thrombophlebitis was markedly high for the infusions of fructose–glucose, antibiotics and anticoagulants or a combination of these three (Table 7.4).

Seven (12%) cannulae fulfilled the criteria for good care and handling, 22 (37%) for less good and 31 (52%) for unsatisfactory to very unsatisfactory (Table 7.5). Significantly more cases of thrombophlebitis were observed in the group whose cannulae were classified as unsatisfactory and very unsatisfactory ($P < 0.01$) (Table 7.5). The level of caring and handling

**Table 7.5**  Development of thrombophlebitis (Th) in relation to cannula care for 60 patients from surgery and internal medicine wards.

| Th/care | Degree | Good care | Less good care | Unsatisfactory care | Very unsatisfactory care |  |
|---|---|---|---|---|---|---|
|  |  | 0 | 1 | 2 | 3 |  |
| No complication | 0 | 5 | 11 | 5 | 2 | 23 |
| Light Th | 1 | — | 8 | 4 | 2 | 14 |
| Medium Th | 2 | 2 | 2 | 2 | 5 | 11 |
| Severe Th | 3 | — | — | 2 | 6 | 8 |
| Very severe Th | 4 | — | 1 | 1 | 2 | 4 |
| Total |  | $n = 7$ | 22 | 14 | 17 | 60 |

**Table 7.6** Grade of nursing care in relation to indwelling time for peripheral cannulae for 60 patients from surgery and internal medicine wards (with percentages in parenthesis).

| | Good care | Less good care | Unsatisfactory care | Very unsatisfactory care | Total (%) |
|---|---|---|---|---|---|
| 1 day | 5 (22) | 13 (57) | 3 (13) | 2 (9) | 100 |
| 2–3 days | 2 (7) | 9 (33) | 6 (22) | 10 (37) | 100 |
| 4–7 days | — | — | 5 (50) | 5 (50) | 100 |
| Total | $n = 7$ | 22 | 14 | 17 | |

decreased the longer the cannula remained *in situ* ($P < 0.01$) (Table 7.6). When the cannula was *in situ* more than 24 hours, the 0.8–1.0 mm size cannula, $n = 20$ (48%), (23 thrombophlebitis noticeable) was used to a greater extent than the 1.2–2.0 mm size cannula, $n = 8$ (13%) (6 thrombophlebitis noticeable) ($P < 0.01$).

**Change of cannulae**

No set routines could be registered for the change of cannulae. Those cannulae which had given complications, according to the definition given, were not removed, whether they were used or not. The patients who arrived from intensive care or the theatre clinic could have up to three cannulae unsatisfactorily fixed and not documented on their anaesthetic record.

The presence of *in situ* cannulae or complications was not documented in the patients' records. In the internal medicine wards there was a list of *in situ* cannulae. The registration was erased when the cannula was removed.

After the cannulae had been removed, seven patients (12%) had no symptoms, 13 (22%) had symptoms for two to four days, 28 (47%) for five to nine days, eight (13%) for 10 to 33 days and four (7%) had symptoms for 98 to 160 days (Table 7.7). The symptoms the patients described while the cannula was *in situ* were discomfort, tenderness, pain, ache, itching, touching the intima of the vein, and pricking. Observations included redness, swelling, induration, haematoma, subcutaneous swelling, nasty-smelling infection and/or red string along the inside of the arm and difficulty in working normally with that arm.

Patients also described that they could feel and follow a hard chord in the vein along the inside of the arm. Afterwards the patients reported discomfort, pricking, pain and difficulty in using a wrist-watch, difficulty in resting the arm against the table because of electric shocks in the vein and difficulty in working normally with that arm.

**Table 7.7**   Number of complication days for the most affected of the 60 patients investigated from surgery and internal medicine wards where day of removal, cannula size, drugs used, number of complication days, age, sex, degree of thrombophlebitis (Th) and degree of care is put into relation.

| Day of removal | Cannula size (mm) | Drug solutions | No. of complication days | Age | Sex | Degree of Th/care | |
|---|---|---|---|---|---|---|---|
| 4 | 1.0 | Rehydrex/antibiotics | 7 | 77 | M | 2 | 3 |
| 4 | 1.2 | Fructose–glucose | 7 | 81 | F | 2 | 2 |
| 4 | 1.2 | Blood | 8 | 80 | M | 2 | 3 |
| 6 | 1.0 | Furix | 9 | 70 | M | 2 | 3 |
| 6 | 1.0 | Anticoagulants/rehydrex | 9 | 60 | M | 3 | 3 |
| 3 | 0.8 | Fructose–glucose | 1 | 70 | M | 3 | 3 |
| 2 | 2.0 | Fructose–glucose | 11 | 80 | F | 3 | 2 |
| 5 | 1.0 | Anticoagulants | 11 | 37 | F | 1 | 2 |
| 8 | 1.0 | Antibiotics | 12 | 67 | F | 3 | 3 |
| 2 | 1.2 | Rehydrex | 12 | 58 | M | 3 | 3 |
| 6 | 1.0 | Fructose–glucose | 16 | 73 | M | 2 | 2 |
| 6 | 1.0 | Antibiotics | 24 | 73 | M | 3 | 3 |
| 5 | 1.2 | Antibiotics | 33 | 31 | M | 2 | 3 |
| 2 | 1.2 | Fructose–glucose/intralipid | 98 | 38 | F | 4 | 2 |
| 6 | 1.0 | Fructose–glucose/ anticoagulants/reomacrodex | 108 | 62 | M | 4 | 3 |
| 3 | 1.0 | Glucose 5% | 150 | 40 | M | 4 | 3 |
| 3 | 1.2 | Fructose–glucose | 150 | 73 | F | 4 | 2 |

M, male; F, female.

**Follow up**

After the hospital stay, 17 patients (28%) were followed up, by means of regular telephone contact because of remaining complications arising from reported symptoms. In these cases, symptoms were noted for two to 150 days (Md = 12) (Table 7.7).

*Discussion*

The purpose of the present study was to describe the frequency of thrombophlebitis related to cannulae location, size, time *in situ*, the care and handling and the duration of the symptoms. In this study, the location of the cannula, as well as the patient's own experience of having a cannula, have been observed and documented daily at the hospital. Only one cannula has been observed in all patients. After discharge, the patients who complained because of symptoms from the cannula location have been followed up, by means of regular telephone calls, until the insertion area, the insertion point and the hand/arm can be said to be free from pain. In order to minimize interrater variability, the observations were carried out by the same person, using fixed variables such as the size of the cannula, fixation, location, medication and solutions, symptoms, frequency, care and handling, documentation and the patient's own experience.

In the current study, one-third of the cannulae used were 1.2 mm (18 gauge) or larger. In the surgery ward, significantly more of the larger cannulae were used, probably because of the possible need for massive infusions in connection with the operation. According to Spanos (1976); Hecher *et al.* (1976), Hecher (1980) and Mossberg (1986, 1988), a 0.8 mm cannula (22 gauge) is completely sufficient for the administration of the most common amount of fluid per day (1–3 litres). Hessov (1981) maintains that it must be an advantage to use a small cannula size with a good infusions flow, and to mix as rapidly as possible with vein blood so as not to damage or irritate the walls intima.

## Unsatisfactorily fixed cannulae

In this study, as in previous studies (MacFarlane *et al.*, 1980; Maki & Band, 1981), the majority of the cannulae were placed on the upper side of the hand. Jones & Craig (1972) found a significantly lower frequency of infusions-related thrombophlebitis in veins on the upper side of the hand compared with the forearm. Other investigations have not shown any significant differences, in frequencies, between different locations (Martin, 1965; Thomas *et al.*, 1970, Asbjörnsen, 1971. They were all well fixed the first day, but when the fixation loosened later nothing was done. The unsatisfactorily fixed cannulae have to be related to the increased risk of infections and development of thrombophlebitis (von Dardel *et al.*, 1986; Hedstrand & Zaren, 1989). Patients who returned from intensive care or the theatre clinic could have up to three cannulae which were unsatisfactorily fixed, although only one was in use. The other cannulae were most likely intended for use during the operation only. Then, owing to an oversight, they accompanied the patient to the medical ward.

During the observation, an increased frequency of complications such as redness, increased discomfort and pain, nasty-smelling infection and purulent insertion site was registered. The symptoms occurred more and more frequently, up to the third day, in 65% of the cases. Thirty-seven (62%) of the cannulae *in situ* caused thrombophlebitis of different degrees. For the patients with the cannula *in situ* for up to 24 hours, the frequency of the thrombophlebitis was significantly lower than for the other patients.

The study has shown that complications and thrombophlebitis increased with time after the insertion of the cannula and markedly after 24 hours. When the cannulae were *in situ* for more than five days and nights (120 hours) all patients ($n = 6$) had thrombophlebitis. This result agrees with earlier studies both nationally and internationally (Skajja *et al.*, 1961; Norell *et al.*, 1972; Collins *et al.*, 1975; Hessov *et al.*, 1977). At the time the study was carried out, there were directives, in the Nursing Manual, that the cannulae were to be removed after 24–48 hours. Furthermore, the logical consequence of the symptoms ought to be that the cannula should have been removed when signs of complications were observed (Maki *et al.*, 1978; von Dardel *et al.*, 1986).

Patients with a peripheral cannula complained of symptoms both during the time the cannula was *in situ* and after. Complications such as redness, swelling, pain, infiltration, induration, haematoma, subcutaneous swelling, nasty-smelling infection or red string along the inside of the arm up to the shoulder were observed in 37 patients (62%). This was considered as different degrees of thrombophlebitis and 20% were said to have severe or very severe thrombophlebitis. Some patients had symptoms for a very long time and complained, in addition to discomfort and pain, that they could feel and follow a hard chord in the vein, along the inside of the arm.

von Dardel *et al.* (1986) and Mossberg (1986, 1988) have shown that thrombophlebitis can arise from 12 to 24 hours, but does not usually appear until two to six days, and can even appear up to 14 days later according to Maddox & Rush (1977). This shows that the irritation in the vein can begin long before it is observed by the nurse. Fonkalsrud *et al.* (1971) and Hessov (1981) point out that thrombophlebitis in deeper lying veins is easier to miss and more difficult to diagnose. In this study, patients without symptoms were not followed up after removal of the cannulae. Some of these may later have developed thrombophlebitis that has not been registered, which can mean that there is a higher frequency than stated here.

### Decreased level of care

The level of the care and handling decreased with the number of days the cannula was *in situ*. After the second day, deficient care and handling were observed. In total, only seven of the 60 patients were estimated to have been correctly handled.

In many cases the nurses had not checked, removed or changed the cannula when it was necessary. The handling did not lead to the removal of the cannula either when redness, tenderness or pain occurred, and the patients' symptoms were not mentioned in the record. Irritating drugs, such as antibiotics, were given in an already tender and swollen vein and those cannulae that were not used were left in place despite the treatment being finished.

Actions that can reduce the frequency of symptoms and thrombophlebitis are good technique, careful hygienic practices (MacFarlane *et al.*, 1980, 1981; Smallman *et al.*, 1980), a small short cannula left *in situ* for less than 24 hours

(Collins *et al.*, 1975, Norell *et al.*, 1972), a well-fixed cannula (von Dardel *et al.*, 1986; Hedstrand & Zaren, 1989) and the avoidance of hypo- or hypertonic solutions (Maki & Martin, 1975; Hessov *et al.*, 1977; Hessov, 1985; Wildsmith, 1978; Brismar & Nyström, 1986). A standardised guide line for management of IV cannulae in the daily care, guarantees these actions (Dudrick *et al.*, 1972; Ryan *et al.*, 1974, Maki & Ringer, 1991).

When treatment and care are given, a patient record should be filled in, according to current laws in Sweden. The notes should be the support and basis for considering the measures, supervision and controls that should be observed. In no case was there any documentation about the inserted cannulae or their complications in the patient's record. This was also true of patients returning from the operating theatre with one or more cannulae still *in situ*. The documentation of the peripheral cannula facilitates the daily observation of the patient's cannula, allowing suitable measures to be taken, which can decrease long and unnecessary pain and suffering for the patient.

## No fixed routines

Fixed routines for insertion, care and handling, removal or documentation of the cannula could not be observed in the actual wards. In the present study, the patients were observed until they were free from symptoms from the cannulation. This extended observation shows that complications caused by peripheral cannulae can be very protracted. In this research study, the patients were followed for up to five months. After the hospital stay, 17 patients were followed up by means of regular telephone contact for two to 150 days (Md = 12) before the insertion area and hand/arm were free from symptoms. This should be seen in relation to current laws, the nurse's responsibility and the quality of the care given to the patient.

## *Conclusion*

Many of the patients displayed their first symptoms on the second day, but the cannula was not removed. Cannulae which are left in the patient's arm/hand in a site which is already irritated cause the patient's symptoms to increase.

The aspects to which a nurse should pay attention in order to ensure good quality of care are: the length of time it is *in situ*, a good fixation and to be well trained in the management of I.V. cannulae so as to avoid complications. The cannula seemed not to be checked regularly and its presence was not documented. Such documentation reminds the nurse on duty that the patient has a cannula which ought to be taken care of correctly so as to avoid protracted complications.

In contrast to the studies previously referred to, this study not only observed the patients during their stay in hospital but even followed them up for some time after their discharge.

## Acknowledgement

Part of this research was supported by the Cancer Foundation, Stockholm, and the Swedish organization for Kidney Diseases, Stockholm. SSF, Swedish Nurses' Association, Stockholm, and Viggo-Spectramed, Helsingborg, Sweden, are also gratefully acknowledged.

## References

Asbjörnsen, G. (1971) Thrombophlebitt og infeksjon ved bruk af plastinfusjonskanyler (in Danish). *Nordisk Medicin*, **86**, 588–92.

Bergqvist, D. (1971) Phosphate buffers in infusion solutions: effects on thrombophlebitis frequency (in Swedish). *Nordisk Medicine*, **86**, 1098–1100.

Brismar, B. & Nyström, B. (1986) Thrombophlebitis and septicemia complications related to intravascular devices and their prophylaxis: a review. *Acta Chirugica Scandinavica*, **530** (suppl.), 73–7.

Buxton, A.E., Highsmith, A.K., Gardner, J.S., West, M., Stamm, W., Dixton, R. *et al.* (1979) Contamination of intravenous infusions fluid: effect of changing administration sets. *Annals of Internal Medicine*, **90**, 764–8.

Collins, C., Collins, J., Constable, F.L. & Johnston, I.D.A. (1975) Infusions thrombophlebitis and infection with various cannulae. *Lancet*, **ii**, 150–53.

von Dardel, O., Mossberg, T. & Svensson, B. (1986) *Insertion of catheters with the accent on peripheral veins* (in Swedish). Anaesthesic clinic, St Görans hospital. Dalbäck & Berglunds printers, Stockholm.

Dudrick, S.J., MacFadyen, B.D., van Buren, C.T., Ruberg, R.L. & Maynard, A.T. (1972) Parenteral hyper alimentation – metabolic problems and solutions. *Annals of Surgery*, **176**, 259–64.

Fonkalsrud, E.W., Carpenter, K., Masuda, J.Y. & Beckerman, J.H. (1971) Prophylaxis against post-infusions phlebitis. *Surgery Gynaecol Obstetric*, **133**, 253–6.

Hamory, B.H. (1987) Nosocomial bloodstream and intravascular device-related infections. In *Prevention and Control of Nosocomial Infections* (ed. R.P. Wenzel), pp. 283–319. Williams & Wilkins, Baltimore.

Hästbacka, J., Tammisto, T., Elfing, G. &Tiitinen, P. (1966) Infusion thrombophlebitis. *Acta Anaesthetica Scandinavica*, **10**, 9–30.

Hecher, J.F. (1980) Thrombus formation on cannulae. *Anaesthesia and Intensive Care*, **2**, 187–9.

Hecher, J.F., Fisk, G.C. & Farell, P.C. (1976) Measurement of thrombus formation on intravascular catheters. *Anaesthesia and Intensive Care*, **4**, 225–31.

Hedstrand, U. & Zaren, B. (eds) (1989) *Intensive Care Compendium* (in Swedish). Anaesthesic clinic, Academic Hospital, Uppsala, Sweden. Upplands Grafiska AB, Uppsala.

Hessov, I. (1981) Intravenous administration of glucose and fructose in the uncomplicated postoperative period. *Danish Medical Bulletin*, **2**(28) 45– 60.

Hessov, I. (1985) Prevention of infusion thrombophlebitis. *Acta Anaesthetica Scandinavica*, **29**, 33–7.

Hessov, I., Allen, J., Arendt, K. & Gravholt, L. (1977) Infusions thrombophlebitis in a surgical department. *Acta Chirurgica Scandinavica*, **143**, 151– 4.

*International Classification of Diseases* (1986) ninth rev. (Swedish version). Liber Allmänna Förlag, Stockholm.

Jones, M.V. & Craig, D.B. (1972) Venous reaction to plastic intravenous cannulae. Influence of cannula composition. *Canada Anaesthetic Soc. Journal*, **19**(49) 1–497.

Lodge, J.P.A., Chisholm, E.M. Breunan, T.G. & Macfie, J. (1987) Insertion technique, the key to avoid infusion phlebitis: a prospective clinical trial. *British Journal of Clinical Practice*, **41**(7), 816–19.

MacFarlane, J.T., Ward, M.J., Banks, D.C., Pilkington, R. & Finch, R.G. (1980) Risk from cannulae used to maintain intravenous access. *British Medical Journal*, **281**, 1395–6.

MacFarlane, J.T., Ward, M.J., Banks, D.C., Pilkington, R. & Finch, R.G. (1981) Reducing risk from intravenous cannulae. *British Medical Journal*, **282**, 1838.

Maddox, R.R. & Rush, D.R. (1977) Double blind study to investigate methods to prevent cephalothin induced phlebitis. *American Journal of Hospital Pharmacy*, **34**, 29–34.

Maki, D.G., & Band, J.D. (1981) A comparative study of polyolyantibiotic and iodophor ointments in prevention of vascular catheter related infection. *American Journal of Medicine*, **70**, 739–44.

Maki, D.G. & Martin, W.T. (1975) Nationwide epidemic of septicemia caused by contaminated infusion products. IV: Growth of microbial pathogens in fluids for intravenous infusion. *Journal of Infectious Diseases*, **131**, 267–72.

Maki, D. & Ringer, M. (1991) Risk factors for infusion-related phlebitis with small peripheral venous catheter. *Annals of Internal Medicine*, **114**, 845–54.

Maki, D.G., Goldman, D.A. & Rhame, F.S. (1978) Infection control in intravenous therapy. *Annals of Internal Medicine*, **79**, 867–87.

Martin, J.T. (1965) Plastic devices for intravascular therapy. *Anaesthetic & Analgetic Journal*, **44**, 25–9.

Mossberg, T. (1981) *Completely Intravenous Nutrition* (in Swedish). Dahlbergs & Co., Stockholm.

Mossberg, T. (1986, 1988) *Technique of Parenteral Nutrition in Peripheral Veins*. Report of study from St Görans Hospital. Lecture on TPN-Days, Stockholm.

Nordenström, J., Jeppson, B., Loven, L. & Larsson, J. (1991) Peripheral parenteral nutrition: effect of a standardized compounded mixture on infusion phlebitis. *British Journal of Surgery*, **78**, 1391–4.

Norell, K., Morgensen, L., Nyqvist, O. & Orinius, E. (1972) Thrombophlebitis following intravenous Lignocain infusion. *Acta Medicin Scandinavica*, **192**, 262–5.

*Pharmaceutical Specialities in Sweden* (FASS) (1991) (ed. A.-G. Hedstrand) Linfo Läkemedelsinformation AB, Stockholm.

Ryan, J.A., Abel, R.M., Abbott, W.M., Hopkins, C.C., Chensey, T., Colley, R., Philips, K. & Fischer, J.E. (1974) Catheter complications in total parenteral nutrition. *New England Journal Medicine*, **290**, 757–61.

Skajja, T., Dahl, J., Kaalund-Jensen, J. & Kvisselgaard, N. (1961) The frequency of thrombophlebitis after intravenous infusion (in Danish). *Nordisk Medicin*, **66**, 1447–51.

Smallman, L.A., Burdon, D.W. & Alexander-Williams, J. (1980) The effect of skin preparation and care on the incidence of superficial thrombophlebitis. *British Journal of Surgery*, **67**, 861–2.

Spanos, H.G. (1976) Thrombus formation on indwelling venous cannulae in sheep: effects of time, size and material. *Anaesthetic and Intensive Care*, **4**, 217–24.

Spanos, H.G. & Hecher, J.F. (1979) Effects of heparine, aspirine and dipyridamole on thrombus formation on venous catheters. *Anaesthetic and Intensive Care*, **7**, 244–47.

Thomas, E.T., Evers, W. & Racz, G.B. (1970) Post infusion phlebitis. *Anaesthetic & Analgetic Journal*, **49**, 150–59.

Wildsmith, J. (1978) Techniques of intravenous infusion. *Scottish Medical Journal*, **23**, 298–306.

# Chapter 8
# Patients' experience of technology at the bedside: intravenous infusion control devices

S. DIANNE PELLETIER, *RN, BScN (Can), DipEdNsg (Sydney),*
*BEdStudies (Qld), MSciSoc (NSW)*
Senior Lecturer, Center for Graduate Nursing Studies, University of Technology,
Sydney, New South Wales, Australia

Within health care systems, rapid and pervasive technological development is occurring with significant ramifications for both nurses and patients. In order to determine the patient's perception of the experience of clinical equipment at the bedside, an exploratory study of 150 hospitalized patients was undertaken. For this study an item of electronic clinical 'hardware', the infusion control device, used increasingly by nurses, was selected as an exemplar of bedside nursing technology. A positive patient response to the equipment and its management was found. The majority of respondents understood the reasons for the equipment's use, were not disturbed greatly by the alarms, had few concerns about the equipment and would welcome further use. A majority felt that the care they received was more patient centred than technology centred. Several recommendations for nursing practice follow from these findings.

## Increasing levels of technology

Increasing levels of technology in the acute care system have considerable potential to affect the patient and his personal human experience of illness, which is crucial to the focus of nursing. As professionals, nurses must develop a keen interest in health care technology and the effect of its usage on their patients. Such an interest is fundamental to the holistic focus of nursing. Nurses are taught to view the patient as a whole person and must be aware of the importance of:

'assessing variations in the complexity, familiarity, comfort, and value that may be concurrently occurring for each participant... It is critical that nurses view the complexity and familiarity, the high and the low of technology, not only as clinicians but also from the patient's and family's viewpoint.'

Carnevali (1985)

Increased understanding of the impact of seemingly 'ordinary' equipment will assist the nurse to consider actual and potential, positive and negative effects on the patient of clinical equipment at the bedside and to incorporate such devices into their patient care more optimally. 'Only a limited amount of research has been conducted on the ... triad of technology, patient and the nurse' (Pillar *et al.*, 1990). Nursing has taken a reactive rather than proactive role in the introduction and assessment of technology and more active nursing participation would be desirable (Braun *et al*, 1984; Pillar *et al.*, 1990; McConnell, 1992, 1993; Pelletier, 1990).

## The study

In order to increase understanding of the patient's technological experience, this study was undertaken to explore hospitalized patients' experience of infusion control devices (ICDs) used in intravenous therapy. The specific objectives were to explore patients' understanding of the ICD, the source of the explanation, their fears, concerns and degree of comfort with the ICD and their perception of the focus of nursing attention. The relationship of the ICD to their feelings of safety and level of illness and their feelings in response to alarms and other mechanical noises were determined.

The presence of the intravenous infusion itself has a primary impact on the patient's activities. A secondary effect may be felt if the ICD makes the patient even less mobile or independent. This can occur if the portable pole is harder to push with the ICD attached, if it is clamped to the bed itself or if the patient is reluctant to unplug it and use the battery. ICD use may result in the use of shorter tubing which can reduce patient movement and freedom. The awkwardness of manipulating tubing through sleeves may contribute to less complete patient dressing. A device that alarms frequently may become a disruptive environmental feature.

### Impact on patient

ICDs, both pumps and controllers, were selected to represent nursing controlled, bedside, technological equipment in clinical (non-intensive care) use which has the potential to affect the aware patient. The numbers of ICDs used are increasing rapidly in general hospital wards as hospital stays are becoming shorter and the hospital population is generally in the more acute phase of their health problem (Golonka, 1986; McConnell, 1991). Acutely ill patients are being increasingly placed in general wards of the hospitals rather than in specialized critical care units.

ICDs, once almost exclusively the province of speciality areas such as intensive or coronary care or neonatal units, are now increasingly found in general wards for administration of total parenteral nutrition, narcotic, cytotoxic and other drug infusions. The increasing tendency for nurses to desire or demand ICDs is also acknowledged (Brewer, 1983; Hamilton, 1984).

ICDs are managed by nurses, to a large extent, and therefore the impact becomes largely an area of nursing responsibility and interest. Unlike many other machines, ICDs are in close contact with the patient 24 hours a day, increasing the potential to have a significant impact. There can be a tendency to overlook the fact that the patient may not be as comfortable with this electronic equipment as the practitioner. Although the hospital and tools are familiar to the nurse, both may appear threatening or at least puzzling and become a source of stress to the patient and family (Benner & Wrubel, 1989; Wilson, 1991). The nurse has a major role in making this foreign environment feel safe and even healing to the patient and the family (Benner & Wrubel, 1989; Pelletier, 1990).

## *Literature review*

Examination of the literature shows that the majority focuses on the equipment itself in terms of design, mechanical operation and uses (Bivans *et al.*, 1980; Kelly & Christensen, 1983; Beaumont, 1987), the selection of the correct device and development of protocols (Kitrenos *et al*, 1978; Alexander *et al.*, 1987), the cost-effectiveness (Bivans *et al.*, 1980; Hoffman *et al.*, 1981; Alexander, 1987), or the accuracy of the devices (Turco, 1978; Yates, 1983; Alexander, 1987; Runciman *et al.*, 1987). Safety aspects such as consistency of flow, electrical faults and air embolism are explored. Most concerns such as these have been significantly reduced by improved technology and increasingly sophisticated alarm systems. As electronic equipment they are relatively safe: however, if misused or faulty, patient injury can occur.

A small proportion of the literature on ICDs relates to psychosocial aspects and the patient's personal experience which is the focus of this study. Turco (1978), Rapp *et al.* (1979) and Hoffman *et al.* (1981) consider the effect on the patient in terms of increased use of the intravenous site, reduced phlebitis and better vein care. Kelly & Christensen (1983) include reduced morbidity. Engler & Engler (1986) consider patient comfort in terms of infiltration, occlusion, phlebitis necessitating re-insertion. These works still focus on the treatment and cost-effectiveness rather than the quality of the patient's experience.

Consideration of the effect of the ICD on the quality of the personal experience is implied by Kitrenos *et al.* (1978) in their recommendation for longer lines to increase ability to move. If the pump reduces mobility it is noteworthy. It is time-consuming and awkward to pass intravenous lines, especially with dedicated pump cartridges, through clothing. Kitrenous *et al.* also acknowledge that the devices are often at the bedside of anxious patients and that there is a need to reduce mechanical pump noises.

### Stress and anxiety levels

Carlquist (1981) claims that a patient's stress and anxiety levels almost inevitably rise, in some cases to extreme levels, with both the anticipation and insertion of an I.V. cannula. It is likely that re-insertion will have a similar and perhaps more profound effect, dependent partly upon the quality of the previous experience. Whether patients believe that they are safer with an ICD or that it may help to preserve their drip site (avoiding re-insertion) could have an effect on their level of stress. Patients may react negatively to I.V. insertion and infusion because they are fearful that they must remain in bed and lose independence and control of activities of daily living (Carlquist, 1981).

The level of anxiety or dissatisfaction can relate to the level of understanding or the quality of explanation given. Sartain (1983) suggests that patients are dissatisfied about the amount of information they receive about their intravenous therapy.

## *The tool*

A 22-item questionnaire of single-response multiple-option closed questions was developed. Questions were designed to explore five central themes which are listed below.

### Patients' understanding of the ICD

Seven questions related to the patients' understanding of the purpose of the ICD, the source of explanation and accuracy of their perception of its cost. Two inter-related questions ascertained whether the patient understood the reason for the intravenous therapy and subsequent ICD usage. For example, a patient might indicate that their I.V. was to administer drug therapy such as heparin and the ICD was used to control the speed of the drug delivery. The accuracy of their perception was determined by the researcher who established with the ward staff why the patient had an I.V. and ICD in use prior to approaching the patient. The source of explanations regarding the equipment and whether more information was wanted were identified.

### Fears, concerns and degree of comfort with the ICD

Patients were asked if they were concerned about mechanical breakdown, overly rapid infusions, mobility restriction, air bubbles or electrical risks. Their perception of what would happen if the device failed and the alarm did not sound was determined. Options available ranged from nothing serious to the need for re-siting or air embolism. Their willingness to press buttons on the machine was felt to indicate an element of their feeling of control over the machine and their relationship to it.

### Perceived relationship of the ICD to illness and safety

Patients were asked if they felt safer or less safe with the ICD in use and whether they felt that patients with an ICD were sicker or less sick than those who did not have ICDs. The term 'sicker' was taken to mean that, in the layperson's perception, the individual was more seriously ill and needed the technological support of the ICD. Patients were asked if they would wish to have the machine again in any future intravenous experience; this response had potential implications for their expectation of care and for health resources.

### Response to alarms and noises

Patients were asked about the frequency of ICD alarms over 24 hours and at night, and their responses to both. These four questions were designed to determine whether the alarms are disturbing to patients.

### Perceived focus of nursing attention.

In order to establish the patients' perception of the focus of care, the perceived frequency of the nurse checking the intravenous equipment and the intravenous site and where they felt the focus of care to be, were determined. The frequency of the nurse giving an explanation for alarms sounding was included.

## Sampling and survey procedure

The questionnaire was piloted on a sample of 10 patients and minor changes made. Subsequently, 156 respondents were surveyed. Since the questionnaires were distributed and collected on an individual basis, a response rate of 95% was achieved. The sample consisted of 150 hospital patients in general medical surgical wards in a 780-bed university teaching hospital (97 responses), a 220-bed public hospital (21 responses) and a 110-bed private hospital (32 responses). There was no distinction made between the respondents from different institutions. Data were collected over a nine-month period.

Subjects were selected from the pool of patients with ICDs in use according to their availability at the time of the researcher's visit, making this essentially a convenience sample. Patients within intensive care units were excluded from the survey as it was felt the additional technological equipment in these areas would alter their perception of the impact of the ICD itself.

Subjects were required to be 18 years of age or over, speak English and to have had over 12 hours' experience of the ICD at the time of completing the questionnaire. Patients who had had the ICD use discontinued within the three hours prior to completing the questionnaire were also included.

## Bias

There were a series of factors which affected the sample selection and led to a biased sample. Patients who were occupied with treatments or care activities, sleeping, involved with visitors or out of the ward would not have been approached at that time. Patients who were identified by the nursing unit manager or ward staff as confused or heavily sedated (often by narcotic infusion) were excluded. Refusal of access by staff occurred once and recommendation against access occurred eight times. A total of seven patients expressed an unwillingness to participate.

The nursing unit manager or other registered nurse was first approached to confirm that it was appropriate to approach the patient. A brief explanation of the study was given to the patient and the researcher determined that the patient understood what was meant by the terms 'intravenous' or 'drip' and 'pump'. The explanation was complemented by the introductory page of the questionnaire. Written consent was obtained from each patient in the large hospital but was not required by the administration of the others as consent was taken to be implicit in the completion of the paper.

The questionnaire was completed at that time or left with the patient, collected later or returned through the internal mail system. Alternatively, several patients expressed willingness to complete the questionnaire but felt unable either to read it or to write. For these patients (16) the researcher read the questions and answers and marked the selected responses. No extra explanations or discussion were given and these responses were not separated from the others. No tests were done to determine if the responses of this group differed from written ones.

## *Results*

The sample was 46% female and 54% male; 35% were between 36 and 55 years and 41% between 56 and 75 years of age. There were no age or sex related differences in relation to the areas studied.

### Understanding purpose of device

Responses reflecting understanding of the purpose of the device by the majority (85%) of respondents and the level of satisfaction (73%) with the information offered is presented in Table 8.1 in relation to the members of the health care team who gave the explanations. A total of 59% identified nursing staff as the source of explanation and 20% identified a medical doctor. Fifteen per cent of respondents were correct in their understanding of the device use, although they indicated that they had not had an explanation. Despite 21% indicating that they had had no explanation, 73% were satisfied with their level of information while 18% wanted to know more.

Of the 21% without explanation, 15% claimed to have no significant worries and 15% were correct in their understanding of why the ICD was being used. This group had a higher rate of 4% for the 'do not know' option relating to the reason why the ICD was in use.

There were no differences in the level of understanding displayed by patients receiving explanations from different sources. Of the 21% who felt that they had not had an explanation, only 6% indicated that they would like more information than they had received and 14% were content with the information that they had.

**Table 8.1**   Understanding and source of explanation (*n* = 150) (in percentages).

|  | Registered nurse | Nurse unit manager | Doctor | No one | Total |
|---|---|---|---|---|---|
| Understanding of ICD use |  |  |  |  |  |
| Correct | 26 | 26 | 18 | 15 | 85 |
| Incorrect | 3 | 3 | 2 | 2 | 10 |
| Do not know | 0 | 1 | 0 | 4 | 5 |
| Total | 29 | 30 | 20 | 21 | 100 |
| Desire for information |  |  |  |  |  |
| More | 7 | 3 | 2 | 6 | 18 |
| Less | 2 | 5 | 1 | 1 | 9 |
| Same | 19 | 23 | 17 | 14 | 73 |
| Total | 28 | 31 | 20 | 21 | 100 |

**Table 8.2**  Feelings of safety in relation to the ICD (*n* = 150) (in percentages).

|  | Safer | Less safe | No difference | Total |
|---|---|---|---|---|
| **Greatest worry** |  |  |  |  |
| Nil | 34 | 0 | 22 | 56 |
| Pump air in | 6 | 0 | 3 | 9 |
| Reduces mobility | 9 | 2 | 9 | 20 |
| Mechanical failure | 8 | 1 | 3 | 12 |
| Other | 0 | 0 | 1 | 1 |
| Total | 57 | 3 | 38 | 98 |
| **Expectation if ICD fails and alarm does not sound** |  |  |  |  |
| Nil | 33 | 2 | 14 | 49 |
| Pump air in | 4 | 1 | 2 | 7 |
| Stop/block/need re-siting | 5 | 1 | 10 | 15 |
| Not known | 16 | 1 | 13 | 29 |
| Total | 58 | 5 | 39 | 100 |
| **Feeling regarding air in line** |  |  |  |  |
| Indifferent | 64 | 46 |  |  |
| Concerned | 75 | 54 |  |  |

## Patients' concerns

The data on the patients' concerns are shown in relation to their feelings of safety (Table 8.2). Fifty-seven per cent felt safer with the device in use, whereas 38% felt no difference in terms of safety. Of the 3% who felt less safe, mobility disruption was the primary concern. Just over half (56%) claimed to have no worries regarding the ICD. Only 9% of respondents identified the potential for air to be accidentally pumped into them and 54% indicated that air in the line concerned them. The disruption of mobility was a concern for 20% and mechanical breakdown for 4%.

A question about expectations of the result of an ICD failure without the alarm sounding led to the emergence of a different pattern from that of the question of major concern. A percentage of 49 thought that there would be no serious effects as the nurse would react to the alarm eventually and 29% responded that they did not know what would happen.

Table 8.3 shows the data relating to the impact of the ICD on the patient's perception of safety and seriousness of illness in relation to the source of the explanation. Percentages of response in relation to thinking those with the device are sicker and whether it would be desirable to have it again are included in Table 8.3. Fifty-eight per cent of the sample felt safer with the ICD in use, with only 4% feeling less safe. However, 44% felt that those receiving ICD therapy were sicker.

The patients' expression of feeling safer, less safe or no different in relation to the presence of the ICD did not seem to be affected by the presence or

**Table 8.3**  *Perception of safety and illness (n = 150) (in percentages).*

|  | Source of explanation | | | | |
|---|---|---|---|---|---|
|  | Registered nurse | Nurse unit manager | Doctor | No one | Total |
| Feeling of safety |  |  |  |  |  |
| Safer | 12 | 22 | 12 | 12 | 58 |
| Less safe | 1 | 2 | 1 | 0 | 4 |
| No difference | 15 | 8 | 7 | 8 | 38 |
| Total | 28 | 32 | 20 | 20 | 100 |

| Think patients with ICDs are sicker | |
|---|---|
| Yes | 44 |
| No | 56 |

| Desire to have a pump again | |
|---|---|
| Yes | 80 |
| No | 12 |
| Indifferent | 8 |

absence of an explanation or its source. A large majority would wish to have the ICD used in their future care.

## Impact of alarms

Table 8.4 presents the impact of the alarms in relation to the frequency of their occurrence and the resultant feelings and expectations if the alarms failed. A percentage of 46 indicated the ICD alarm had sounded between two and five times in the last 24 hours. An alarm rate of greater than 10 in the previous 24 hours was identified by 12%. Overall, 23% expressed indifference and 49% appreciation, as opposed to negative responses of concern (19%) or annoyance (9%).

Even for those 16% who were often awakened at night, the neutral (24%) or positive (50%) response to the alarms exceeded concern (17%) and annoyance (9%). Those experiencing frequent alarms did not express a greater need for more information than other groups. The explanation or lack of it did not relate to the feelings experienced when an alarm is heard. One-quarter felt that explanations regarding alarms were infrequent. Also 91% of respondents were not disturbed by other noises that ICD devices made.

## Focus of nursing care

Table 8.5 displays data relating to the patients' perception of the focus of nursing care. For 55% of the sample the individual was felt to be the focus,

**Table 8.4**   Impact of the alarms (*n* = 150) (in percentages).

| | Frequency of pump alarm in previous 24 hours | | | | |
|---|---|---|---|---|---|
| | 0–1 | 2–5 | 6–10 | > 10 | Totals |
| Feeling at sounding of alarms | | | | | |
| Indifferent | 4 | 12 | 4 | 3 | 23 |
| Concerned | 3 | 8 | 6 | 2 | 19 |
| Glad it alerts nurse | 17 | 22 | 7 | 3 | 49 |
| Annoyed | 0 | 4 | 1 | 4 | 9 |
| Total | 24 | 46 | 18 | 12 | 100 |
| Expectation if ICD fails and alarm does not sound | | | | | |
| Nil | 10 | 22 | 11 | 5 | 48 |
| Pump air in | 2 | 3 | 1 | 1 | 7 |
| Stop/block/need re-siting | 3 | 8 | 2 | 3 | 16 |
| Not known | 10 | 12 | 4 | 3 | 29 |
| Total | 25 | 45 | 18 | 12 | 100 |

| | Perception of frequency of alarms at night | | | |
|---|---|---|---|---|
| | Rarely | Occasionally | Often | Total |
| Feeling regarding alarms | | | | |
| Indifferent | 8 | 12 | 4 | 24 |
| Concerned | 7 | 6 | 4 | 17 |
| Glad it alerts nurse | 22 | 22 | 6 | 50 |
| Annoyed | 1 | 6 | 2 | 9 |
| Total | 38 | 46 | 16 | 100 |

whereas 37% felt the centre of attention was more on the mechanical aspects. Ten respondents (8%) created a response category to include both the machine and the individual. Technically these responses should be ignored as non-applicable. However, these responses were identified to show the number who chose to create such a category.

The perceived focus of care was not affected by the source of the explanation nor did it relate to feelings of safety. In terms of focus of care there was no difference between the two groups with the highest perceived frequency of site checks.

## Discussion

The most noteworthy findings are the generally positive or at least neutral effect of the ICD experience. The presence of this technological device at the bedside does not seem as threatening or disruptive as may have been

**Table 8.5**   Focus of care ($n = 150$) (in percentages).

|  | Mechanical aspects | Individual | Both* | Total |
|---|---|---|---|---|
| **Frequency i.v. site perceived to be checked** | | | | |
| 1–2 hourly | 2 | 23 | 1 | 26 |
| 3–8 hourly | 16 | 16 | 4 | 36 |
| If complains or alarms | 13 | 11 | 1 | 25 |
| Do not know | 6 | 5 | 2 | 13 |
| Total | 37 | 55 | 8 | 100 |
| **Desire for information** | | | | |
| More | 8 | 9 | 2 | 18 |
| Less | 2 | 6 | 0 | 8 |
| Same | 28 | 39 | 6 | 73 |
| Total | 38 | 54 | 8 | 99 |
| **Feeling of safety** | | | | |
| Safer | 24 | 32 | 5 | 61 |
| Less safe | 1 | 3 | 0 | 4 |
| No different | 15 | 18 | 2 | 35 |
| Total | 40 | 53 | 7 | 100 |

*This was a response created by 13 respondents and as such should be excluded but is included to show number unwilling to discriminate focus.

anticipated. It seems to offer a form of security that is welcomed. The positive dimensions are the numbers of respondents who:

(1)  Understand the reasons for their intravenous therapy and ICD use.
(2)  Feel safer with the ICD.
(3)  Have positive reactions to the alarms.
(4)  Are not disturbed by the other mechanical noises.
(5)  Perceive the focus to be on the individual.
(6)  Do not perceive themselves to be sicker.

However there are aspects revealed that could warrant nursing attention, such as the number who:

(1)  Perceive a lack of explanation.
(2)  Wish for more information.
(3)  Have general concerns about the device.
(4)  Experience > 10 alarms in 24 hours.
(5)  Perceive the focus to be on the mechanical dimensions.
(6)  Feel concerned about air in the line.
(7)  Feel that an explanation is not given for alarms.
(8)  Would wish to have an ICD again.

**No explanation**

It is noteworthy for the nursing and health-related professions that nearly one-quarter of the sample indicated that no one had given them an explanation for the ICD or its purpose. It may be that explanations were given which were not heard or understood, as a result of the patient's physical or psychological condition at the time of commencement of therapy. Technology requires increasing levels of explanations and greater use of interpersonal skills (Clifford, 1986; Pelletier, 1990). The fact that the majority were content with the amount of information they had received is heartening for health professionals. Although the level of understanding was high, this may have been gained from previous experience, overhearing interactions or observing the staff, other patient and equipment or other unknown variables not necessarily related to a staff explanation.

Those wanting more information give support to Sartain's claims (1983) and Carnevali's warning (1985) that nurses must remember the patient's and family's needs in relation to technology. As nurses consider this technological equipment to be within their sphere of practice, it is valuable for them to recognize the opportunity and necessity to use their interpersonal skills to advantage, explaining and interpreting technological equipment that to them is becoming commonplace.

Popular opinion that health care technology will be useful or valuable and non-hazardous (Jennett, 1984; Dorsey 1986) is supported by the majority who would prefer to have an ICD again and by the fact that over half had no significant concerns. This study suggests that technology at the bedside is, for the large majority at least, neutral if not positive in terms of safety and reassurance.

It is perhaps surprising that only 16% of respondents identified the potential for the cannula to block and need re-siting if the pump failed and the alarm did not sound. Yet this is a very legitimate repercussion of pump failure or stoppage. Patients may be experiencing such prompt responses to alarm conditions that they do not perceive blockage as a legitimate concern.

**Alarms**

The level of disturbance to the patients of the potentially disruptive or anxiety-provoking alarms was less than anticipated. Concern is warranted for those experiencing high alarm rates and especially the majority who were awakened at night by the alarms, as the value of sleep to health is recognized. Nursing strategies such as correct selection of devices can reduce the incidence of alarms in many cases. Manufacturers need to be made aware of the overly frequent alarm states and strive for a balance between the need for safety and the sensitivity of the devices.

That a minority were disturbed by other noises may be heartening news for nurses and manufacturers. Some respondents described the grinding or filling noise as comforting and reassuring and some called their machine by a pet name. This suggests patients may personalize technological equipment in a manner similar to that attributed to nurses (Smoyak, 1986; Patterson, 1988).

Nurses may wish to address the question of infrequent explanation of alarms. The nurse may believe that the patient knows why it alarms or is not interested. Furthermore, nurses may not repeat the explanation each time if the reason for the alarm is known and unchanged. However, it is important that the patients understand, if they are able, why the machine alarms in order to alleviate their concerns.

The potential for the device to impede patient mobility (Carlquist, 1981) exists but was not supported by this survey. Mobility disruption was included with other critical options and possibly not explored optimally. Three patients commented on the difficulty of pushing the stands and the top-heavy nature of the intravenous pole with an ICD attached. The potential for mobility impairment with the negative consequences warrants nursing intervention and further empirical examination.

### Positive experience

The generally positive nature of the experience is further supported as the majority would prefer to have the ICD again, which suggests that they value the technological equipment and do not perceive it in a threatening or negative way. The figures show that, for some, this value does not lie in terms of safety. It could be that these patients were considering accuracy, consistency of infusion rates or alarms to summon the nurse as valuable or desirable without equating these factors to safety.

This finding is important if consumers are likely to become more demanding in terms of quality care and quality outcomes. It is possible that as ICDs are used more, and more patients come to expect or request their use, there could be a significant impact on health care costs. This may be particularly true since the study reveals that only one-quarter of the sample had an accurate perception of the costs of the device.

The proportion (56%) of the population who did not feel that patients with ICDs were sicker may reflect the trend to use more technology in general areas as opposed to 'high tech' environments. The potential for those receiving therapy involving technological 'support' to feel sicker or more needy than others could have negative effects upon their stress levels and influence their behaviour and potentially affect the length of the illness period. While for some the perception of greater severity of illness may be a very accurate perception and not related to factors such as the ICD, the effect of technological hardware at the bedside on stress levels or morbidity patterns warrants further examination.

## Implications for care

That the majority feel care is focused on them is heartening. However, considering the nursing focus of individualized and humanistic care (Henderson, 1985) and the dangers identified in the depersonalization of care arguments (Fagerhaugh *et al.*, 1980, Henderson 1985), it is noteworthy that, with this comparatively commonplace bedside technology, 38% did not feel themselves the focus of care. Nurses should endeavour to capitalize on the technology as a tool to free them to focus on the patient. Strategies to enhance this process could prove a worthwhile focus for further research.

These insights into the patients' technological experience are valuable and nurses can use such knowledge to enhance their patients' hospitalization experience.

## *Acknowledgements*

The author wishes to thank the hospitals and respondents who participated in the study.

## *References*

Alexander, M.R. (1987) Infusion control devices: are they always justified? *Drug Intelligence and Clinical Pharmacy*, **21**(3), 255–7.

Alexander, M.R., Kirking, D.M. & Baron, K. (1987) Utilization of electronic infusion devices in a university hospital. *Drug Intelligence and Clinical Pharmacy*, **21**(7/8), 630–33.

Beaumont, E. (1987) I.V. infusion pumps. *Nursing Management*, **18**(9), 26–32, 95–101.

Benner, P. & Wrubel, J. (1989) *The Primacy of Caring Stress and Coping in Health and Illness.* Addison Wesley, Menlo Park, California.

Bivans, B., Rapp., R., Powers, P., Butler, J. & Haack, D. (1980) Electronic flow control and roller clamp control in intravenous therapy. *Archives of Surgery*, **1**(115), 70–72.

Braun, J., Baines, S., Olson, N., Scruby, L., Manteuffel, C. & Cretilli, P. (1984) The future of nursing: combining humanistic and technological values. *Health Values: Achieving High Level Wellness*, **8**(3), 12–15.

Brewer, A. (1983) *Nurses, Nursing and New Technology: Implications of a Dynamic Technological Environment.* School of Health Administration, University of New South Wales, Kensington, Australia.

Carlquist, K. (1981) Understanding the psychological needs of the patient on I.V. therapy: a stress reducing approach. *National Association of Intravenous Therapy Journal*, **4**(9), 368–70.

Carnevali, D. (1985) Nursing perspective in health care technology. *Nursing Administration Quarterly*, **9**(4), 11–12.

Clifford, C. (1986) Patients, relatives and nurses in a technological environment. *Intensive Care Nursing*, **2**, 67–72.

Dorsey, D.B. (1986) The other health care revolution. *Archives of Pathology and Laboratory Medicine*, **110**(4), 264–8.

Engler, M., & Engler, M. (1986) Comparative evaluation of intravenous therapy regulatory devices. *Heart and Lung*, **15**(3), 262–7.

Fagerhaugh, S., Strauss, A., Suczek, B. & Weiner, C. (1980) The impact of technology on patients, providers and care patterns. *Nursing Outlook*, **28**, November, 666–72.

Golonka, L. (1986) Trends in health care and use of technology by nurses. *Medical Instrumentation*, **20**(1), 9.

Hamilton, J. (1984) Nursing and the scientific revolution. *Australian Nurses Journal*, **14**(3), 41–4.

Henderson, V. (1985). The essence of nursing in high technology. *Nursing Administration Quarterly*, **9**(4), 1 9.

Hoffman, D., Attilio, R., Braun, D., Oberst, M. & Stern, N. (1981) A randomized study of the IVAC 230 infusion controller in a comprehensive cancer center. *The American Journal of Intravenous Therapy and Clinical Nutrition*, **8**(9), 16–18.

Jennett, B. (1984) *High Technology Medicine Benefits and Burdens*. Burgess and Son, Abingdon, Oxfordshire.

Kelly, W. & Christensen, L. (1983) Selective patient criteria for the use of infusion control devices. *The American Journal of Intravenous Therapy and Clinical Nutrition*, **10**(2), 18–21, 25, 29.

Kitrenos, J.G., Jones, M. & McLeod, D. (1978) Comparison of selected intravenous infusion pumps and rate regulators. *American Journal of Hospital Pharmacy*, **35**(30), 304–9.

McConnell, E.A. (1991) Key issues in device use in nursing practice. *Nursing Management*, **2**(11), 32–3.

McConnell, E.A. (1992) Technology assessment: the road to appropriate equipment and care. *Nursing Management*, **23**(6), 64a–h.

McConnell, E.A. (1993) Technology assessment applied: a comparison of ophthalmic diagnostic techniques to detect diabetic retinopathy among Aboriginal people in central Australia. *Contemporary Nurse*, **2**(1), 23–8.

Patterson, J. (1988) Cost containment with goods and services: can nursing contribute? *Confederation of Australian Critical Care Nurses Journal*, **1**(3), 24–8.

Pelletier, D. (1990) Technology marches on: considerations for the nursing profession. *Australian Health Care Review*, **13**(3), 203–10.

Pillar, B., Jacox, A.K. & Redman, B.K. (1990) Technology, its assessment and nursing. *Nursing Outlook*, **38**(1), 16–17.

Rapp, R.P., Bivins, B., McKean, H.E., Powers, P. & Butler, J. (1979) Effects of electronic infusion control on the efficiency, complications and cost of I.V. therapy. *Hospital Formulary*, **11**, 975–82.

Runciman, W.B., Ilsley, A.H., Rutten, A.J., Baker, D. & Fronsko, R.R.L. (1987) An evaluation of intravenous infusion control pumps and controllers. *Anaesthetics and Intensive Care*, **15**, 217–18.

Sartain, B. (1983) Nursing considerations in I.V. therapy. *British Journal of Intravenous Therapy*, **4**, March, 4–7.

Smoyak, S.A. (1986) High tech high touch. *Nursing Success Today*, **3**(11), 9–ICD 16.

Turco, S. (1978) Inaccuracies in the I.V. flow rates and the use of pumps and controllers. *Journal of the Parenteral Drug Association*, **32**(5), 242–8.

Wilson, G. (1991) Technology and stress. *Nursing*, **4**(32), 31–4.

Yates, L. (1983) Technology in nursing. *Nursing Focus*, **11**(12), 8.

# Chapter 9
# The primary-care nurse's dilemmas: a study of knowledge use and need during telephone consultations

TOOMAS TIMPKA, *MD, PhD*
Assistant Professor, Departments of Community Medicine and Computer and Information Science

and ELISABETH ARBORELIUS, *PhD*
Assistant Professor, Department of Community Medicine, Linköping University, Linköping, Sweden

In Sweden (population 8 million) there are 20 million calls every year to receptionist nurses at health-care centres. The aim of this study was, first, to develop a general description of these telephone consultations in terms of the decision-making process and inter-personal communication. Second, the dilemmas that receptionist nurses encounter were to be recorded and analysed. A two-level video method was used. At the first level, a video recording of the consultation was used to draw a 'consultation map'. At the second level, the receptionist nurses reviewed and commented on the video-recording using a 'freeze frame' technique for stimulated recall and the comments were categorized. Analysis of the consultation maps showed that the receptionist nurses focused mainly on tasks related to medical diagnosis and management strategy, with less time spent on the patient's concerns, ideas and expectations. Analysis of the dilemmas showed that medical dilemmas were the most frequent, occurring in two consultations out of three. Dilemmas in the area of interpersonal communication frequently concerned distrust, either in what the patient presented, or in what the patient was said to have understood. The conclusions are that the receptionist nurses were oriented towards medical management, and that they employed an informing rather than counselling strategy. Measures must be considered to support the receptionist nurses in the medical decision-making process. Action research is suggested to apply these results in the development of the work-role of the receptionist nurse.

## *Introduction*

The receptionist nurse at a health-care centre (HC) in Sweden is an example of a nurse in a self-contained work role. The receptionist nurse is the first practitioner in the Swedish health care system that a person with a health problem is supposed to contact, normally through a telephone call. According to Marklund & Bengtsson (1989), there are approximately 20 million such calls per year to HCs in Sweden, which has a population of 8 million. Only between half and one third of these calls, depending on the local routines at the HC, lead to an appointment with a general practitioner (GP). Hence, study of the telephone consultations of receptionist nurses allows observation of a nurse in a modern work role, i.e. with the responsibility to manage independently patients with complex biopsychosocial complaints. The work role has three important characteristics:

(1) High organizational responsibility. The receptionist nurse has the responsibility to decide the level of care required, i.e. to give advice for self-care or to arrange an appointment with a nurse or physician.
(2) High independence. Decision-making is from a 'locus-of-control' point of view (Fisher, 1985) performed independently by the nurse.
(3) Need for interpersonal skills. The consultation tasks challenge the communication skills of the nurse (Kagan, 1985).

While discussing their study of nurses managing simulated patients. Tanner *et al.* (1987) contend, first, that corresponding studies in the practice setting are needed and, second, that models other than the commonly used information processing model (Newell & Simon, 1973) are needed for the analysis.

Cicourel (1987) identifies four levels of framing which characterize decision-making in the practice setting: (1) organizational policies, which guide or sanction decisions; (b) interactional conditions, for instance, body posture, which influence the dialogue between patients and medical personnel; (c) language conditions; and (d) comprehension conditions, which affect the use of schematized knowledge as the latter is influenced by a changing local environment.

Information processing models describe the process of decision-making on the basis of verbal reports of the rules on which the decisions are grounded. Woods (1984) points out three major limitations of these models: poor possibilities for generalization; that the reporting of the process may actually alter the processes used in diagnostic reasoning; and that the results are not readily applicable to developing means for assisting decision-making in complex situations.

**Aim of study**

The aim of this study was two-fold:

(1) To develop a general description of the telephone consultation process by the identification of a 'typical' consultation in the practice setting in terms of the decision-making process and inter-personal communication.
(2) To identify and analyse the dilemmas that receptionist nurses face during these telephone consultations, using a method in which the influence on the consultation is minimized. The term dilemma is also used to indicate perplexing situations, not only structured problems, i.e. well-formed questions.

To achieve these ends, a method is needed where both quantitative and qualitative data are collected. Quantitative data are needed to develop a general description of the consultation. Qualitative, phenomenological data are needed for the analysis of dilemmas, since they are intrinsically sub-jective. Moreover, a qualitative, contextual framing is necessary for the analyses since the study entails verbal interaction in an institutional setting, and since the context of presumed responsibilities, duties and routines is essential for the performance of the nurses' work.

## Methods

A two-level method for data collection was used (Timpka & Arborelius, 1989). At the first level, consultation data were collected from a video recording of the telephone consultation. At the second level, identification and analysis of dilemmas was made possible by letting the nurses review and comment on the video recording using a 'freeze frame' technique. A phenomenological analysis of the review comments was performed to understand the dilemma from the nurses' own perspective (Bogdan & Taylor, 1975). The classification structure used in the analysis is based on Habermas' (1979) general epistemological theory.

**Collection of consultation data**

During the research period, all patients calling the HC under study were informed that their telephone conversation might be recorded for research purposes. The selected nurses were videotaped during one entire work shift and both the nurses' and the patients' voices were recorded onto the video-tape. The reason for contact, diagnoses and management actions were noted by the nurses directly after each call. The patients included in the study were contacted by the research team and informed that the consultation had been recorded and asked if they agreed to participate in the study.

## Collection of review data

The video recording was reviewed by the nurse in two sessions with two members of the research team present. One research team member acted as receiver of comments, while the other research team member acted as secretary. The review setting was arranged as a two-person communication between the receiver and the nurse. Before the start of each session, the nurse was firmly assured that no comments would be forwarded to the patient.

For the first review, instructions were given to 'Stop the tape as many times as you desire to comment'. All comments were audiotaped and logged. For the second review, more specific instructions were given: 'Stop the tape when you feel unsure about how to go on'. After each review, the nurse was asked if she had any additional comment. If so, these final comments were included in the analysis.

## Analysis of consultation data

Using the video recordings, a 'consultation map' (Pendelton *et al.*, 1984) was drawn for each consultation. The map is based on defined tasks that practitioners theoretically should consider during consultations in primary health care. It describes, first, the time spent on patient-dependent task topics, i.e. elucidating the nature and history of the problem, aetiology of the problem, the patient's ideas, concerns and expectations, the effect for the patient of the problem, other continuing problems and risk factors. Second, practitioner-dependent task-topics are mapped, i.e. choice of appropriate action, sharing information with the patient and, finally, involving the patient in the management of the problem.

The activity during every 15-second interval of each consultation was classified with respect to the task that was dealt with. In addition, the total number of shifts of task topics, and shifts between patient- and practitioner-dependent task topics were noted for each consultation. Finally, the typical consultation was identified by matching the individual consultation maps against the median time spent on respective task topics, the average consultation time, and the average number of shifts to choose the best match.

## Analysis of review data

Each comment from the videotape reviews of the consultation was analysed in three steps:

(1) Examination of the whole comment to reconstruct the meaning from the nurse's point of view.
(2) Separation of composite comments into subtopics, so that every comment to be classified only deals with one issue.
(3) Sorting of the elementary comments into the predetermined classification structure (see below).

The comments were divided into new observations (for instance, 'Oh, I was not aware that I speak so fast!'), comments directed towards research team members and not addressing the situation on the videotape, and stimulated recall of the consultation (Fig. 9.1). The stimulated recall comments were split into positive remarks and comments regarding dilemma situations.

The dilemma comments were categorized, according to the type of knowledge needed, into the following classification structure based on Habermas' (1979) epistemological theory:

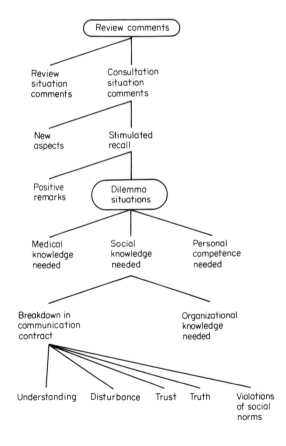

**Fig. 9.1**   The classification schema for review comments. Habermas' (1979) epistemological theory was used for determining the basic categories.

(1) Medical–scientific knowledge.
(2) Social knowledge, divided into knowledge of interpersonal communication and knowledge of social organization.
(3) Personal competence, i.e. knowledge of the nurse's own emotions and opinions, and their role in the interpretation of life events.

The medical–scientific dilemmas were analysed according to occurrence and subject area. For representation of difficulties in interpersonal communication, Habermas' 'claims for valid communication' were used. Thus, communication dilemmas, i.e. situations where the nurse perceived violations of validity claims, were subcategorized into situations where the nurse: did not understand the patient; perceived that the patient violated a social norm; did not trust the patient; disagreed with the patient on the truth of facts; or was disturbed by events in the environment.

The classification was first made independently by the first author, and thereafter validated by the second author. In case of disagreement ( < 5% of the comments), the comment was discussed between the authors and, if necessary, the nurse who gave the comment was contacted.

## Materials

The study was performed at the only HC in a town with 30 000 inhabitants, involving five (of 15) receptionist nurses. All five were female, on average 37 years old (range 31–41 years) and had on average 15 years of experience (range 10–20 years). None of them had special training in communication skills or decision-making. There was no formal introduction for new receptionist nurses at the HC. They were introduced instead by 'sitting beside' experienced colleagues.

The involved nurses were all individually informed about the aims of the study, and were given the possibility to withdraw. A centralized organizational model was used at the HC, as all patient calls were pooled and connected by the telephone exchange operator to the first available nurse. The usual routines at the HC were followed as much as possible while collecting data for the study, and there was no selection of patients.

Thirty-three consultations were scheduled for analysis; 22 managed by the nurse without arranging an appointment with a general practitioner (GP) at the HC, and 11 resulting in a GP consultation. Two patients, one from each category, chose not to participate in the study. Four nurses had six to eight consultations analysed, and one had three consultations.

## Results

The duration of the 31 consultations ranged between 1 min. 25 sec. and 10 min. 00 sec, with he mean being 3 min. 25 sec. According to the nurses' notes, the main reasons why the participating patients contacted the HC were infectious diseases (10 cases) and orthopaedic problems (seven cases). These were followed by problems within internal medicine (three cases), ophthalmology (three cases), surgery (two cases), dermatology (two cases) and miscellaneous problems (four cases). Of the 21 consultations managed by the nurse, six were handled by advising pharmacological treatment, six were taken in to be seen by the nurses, six were given advice and asked to wait and call again if the symptoms did not improve, and three were advised to contact the local hospital.

## Consultation mapping

Of the patient-dependent consultation task topics, nature and history of problems were dealt with in all 31 consultations, aetiology in 17 consultations, the patient's own ideas about the problem in nine consultations, the patient's concerns in 18 consultations, the patients' expectations in four consultations, the effects of the problem in one consultation, continuing problems in three consultations, and risk factors in none of the consultations. Concerning the practitioner-dependent task topics, an explicit action was decided on by the nurse in all 31 consultations, background information relating to the actions chosen was shared with the patient in 25 consultations, and the patient was actively encouraged to be involved in the management of the problems in six consultations.

The median number of task topics dealt with during a consultation was seven, ranging between three and 12 (the same topic could be returned to several times during a consultation). Shifts between patient- and practitioner-dependent task topics (i.e. the nurse shifting between receiving and giving information) occurred a median of three times per consultation, with the range between one and 12. Management action was decided on by the nurse after an average of 1 min. 25 sec. The typical consultation with regard to the above general characteristics is shown in Fig. 9.2.

## Dilemma situations

From 145 review comments, 87 dilemma situations could be distinguished. The situations were categorized into medical–scientific dilemmas (57%), social dilemmas (36%) and dilemmas involving personal competence (7%) (Fig. 9.3).

### Medical–scientific dilemmas

Twenty of the 50 dilemmas involving medical knowledge were diagnostic dilemmas, while 30 dilemmas concerned choice of management strategy.

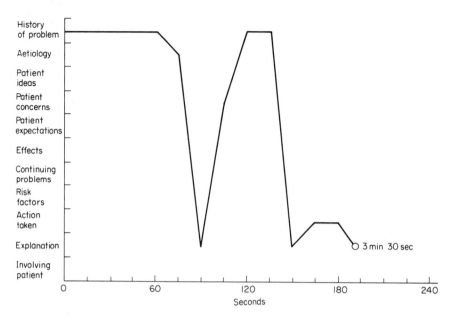

**Fig. 9.2**  Consultation map. A typical telephone consultation in primary care based on: topics covered; number of shifts between topics; and consultation length. The patient was a woman contacting the HC due to pain in her left shoulder. After a short discussion, it became clear that the patient was worried about a breast lump, and wanted a mammography examination. She was advised by the nurse to contact the department of radiology at the local hospital.

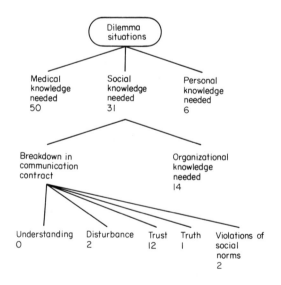

**Fig. 9.3**  The number of comments in each of the categories describing dilemmas. The comments originated from five nurses reviewing video recordings of 31 telephone consultations in primary care.

*Occurrence*

In eight consultations, the nurse faced three medical dilemmas or more, in 12 consultations one or two dilemmas were confronted, while during the remaining 11 consultations no medical dilemmas occurred. Divided into subject areas, dilemmas concerning choice of management strategy occurred in 16 consultations, while diagnostic dilemmas were identified in 14 consultations.

*Subject area*

The most common dilemma in the choice of management strategy was to decide if the patient was to see a GP or not. One patient had been in contact with the outpatient clinic at the hospital one month prior to the consultation because of a minor eye injury, and was calling since he still had symptoms:

'I was carefully thinking over what to do, since I knew how few appointment times [with GPs] we had available here ... and the length of time that had passed between the first time he was at the hospital and now.'

Another frequent management choice concerned pharmacological therapy. The nurses advised patients of non-prescription drugs that they could buy themselves, as well as arranged prescriptions from a GP. In one case, a nurse had difficulties managing a patient with a history of duodenal ulcer:

'Really, I was not sure of what to do. I felt that I had pressed her to accept the Zantac tablets, regardless of whether she wanted them or not ... She accepted them later, all right ... Well, I don't know.'

Concerning diagnosis, the nurses seldom described difficulties with collecting data. The dilemmas occurred instead when conclusions were to be drawn, having formulated the problem. A typical dilemma occurred when a woman called about problems with swallowing:

'It is very hard to know what this can be. It could be anything ... it could be goitre, or something psychiatric, or a tonsillitis, or is it an ordinary virosis, or ... there are lots of alternatives to choose from.'

The consultation ended in the nurse arranging an appointment with a GP.

A special type of diagnostic dilemma involved the telephone counselling situation since the nurse did not see the patient in person. For instance, one nurse described her way of reasoning about a patient with dermatological complaints:

'I tried to imagine what these things look like, almost so that I could see for myself how they look ... They look like this and this and that.'

*Social dilemmas*

The 31 dilemmas classified as social were divided into those caused by: a breakdown in the organizational structure surrounding the consultation (45%); and interruptions during the communication with the patient (55%).

*Organizational breakdown*
Situations where failure in the organizational routines at the HC disrupted the nurse occurred during 11 consultations. The most common situation occurred when the medical record was not available. Other dilemma types that occurred more than once concerned the policy for referral to the local hospital, and lost messages concerning test results for patients received from local GPs and hospital physicians. A typical comment was:

> 'This is a dilemma, when you don't have the medical record handy so that you can give the test result at once! Alright, according to the instructions, we shouldn't give out the results of these tests over the phone ... but it is still normal practice to do so if the tests are OK. Now she has to wait another five days for a letter. Poor patient.'

*Communication dilemmas*
During 10 consultations, 17 situations occurred where the nurse perceived difficulties in the communication with the patient. These dilemmas are divided, according to Habermas' theory, into situations where the nurse: perceived that the patient violated a social norm (two dilemmas), did not trust the patient (12 dilemmas), disagreed with the patient on the truth of facts (one dilemma) or was disturbed (two dilemmas). No comment was made which indicated difficulties in understanding a patient. A situation when a nurse felt that a patient violated a social norm occurred when a patient failed to appear for an appointment. A disagreement on the truth of a fact concerned whether new glasses could be the cause of vertigo. Nevertheless, the most common communication dilemma was not trusting the patient. This occurred when the nurse doubted what the patient actually had said. However, situations also occurred where the nurse had informed the patient, but was still not confident that the patient had understood. Typical comments were:

> 'This is strange! He planned to go to work! If he really had the back pain he described, he ... I decided to not take that discussion. There was no use!'

> 'Funny thing, she was able to go to work in that condition! She worked every night from four to twelve.'

> 'I felt she had problems understanding the information. It is possible that I did not explain well enough.'

*Dilemmas involving personal competence*

During five consultations, six situations occurred where the personal competence of the nurse was challenged. These dilemma situations had to do with the choice of the most practical and convenient way to proceed during a telephone consultation. One nurse commented on a situation which occurred when she came back to a patient after having searched for his medical record:

> 'I said, "Hello again, Johnny!" Maybe I was too personal in this situation. I don't know what he thinks. But I am a spontaneous kind of person, and I want the patients to learn to know me the way that I am, and trust me ... so it doesn't feel like there is a barrier between me and the patient. I want it open like this.'

## Discussion

The consultation-map analysis of the work routines of the receptionist nurses showed an emphasis on tasks related to diagnosis and choice of medical management strategy, with relatively little time spent on patient concerns, ideas and expectations. Previously, Faulkner (1979) also found that nurses' communications with patients are focused on procedural topics. This correlates poorly with the Swedish law on informed consent, i.e. that patients should be involved in all decisions regarding their health care (Swedish Health and Medical Services Act, 1985). Morrison & Burnard (1989) have shown in studies of nurses' interpersonal skills that both student nurses and experienced nurses perceive themselves as more skilful in the use of prescriptive, supportive and informative interventions than in confronting or enabling interventions. Hence, one explanation of the low attention to patients' desires is that the nurses avoid these matters since they perceive themselves less skilful on interventions in this area. However, Fielding & Llewelyn (1987) argue that what may appear to be 'poor communication' may occur because the nurse does not 'want' to communicate well. Therefore, another reason for not focusing on the patient's desires may be lack of time, i.e. nurses simply felt that they did not have time to discuss other less immediate treatment alternatives or to confront patients on controversial issues.

Yet, whichever the reason, the receptionist nurses in the telephone consultations were informing rather than counselling, given that the latter is defined as 'a method of withholding advice, refraining from decision making, exploring feelings, leading the client to discover his own coping mechanism' (Altschul, 1983, cited in Wilson-Barnett, 1988).

The analysis of the consultation dilemmas showed that dilemmas concerning medical reasoning were the most frequent, occurring in two consultations out of three. This frequency of dilemmas is proportional to the consultation content as mirrored by the mapping of task topics. Several studies investigating medical reasoning strategies of nurses using simulated patients have been reported. Holtzemer (1986) observed that nurses are proficient on data collection and focus on choice of therapy, not diagnosis. In the present study, the nurses mainly described difficulties in drawing conclusions from collected data, not in collecting and interpreting data. Slightly more comments concerned choice of therapy than establishing a diagnosis. Hence, it is plausible to assume that, for effectiveness, the receptionist nurses employed an uncomplicated decision strategy (average time to deciding action was 1 min. 25 sec.) and faced difficulties when data did not fit preformed decision models. Some support for this view is also provided by de Graaf (1989), who found, when comparing groups of nurses and physicians, that the nurse group had lower inter-rater decision variability than the physician group. She suggests that this may be due to nurses considering medical problems at a less complex level.

Contextual influence was repeatedly reported by the nurses in this study in dilemmas concerning choice of management alternatives, but not in diagnosis. Dilemmas in management decisions appeared to occur due to situational factors, the most prevalent being the availability of GPs on that day. This finding supports Field (1987) in her view that the decision-making process of nurses in the practice setting is, to a considerable extent, constrained by factors absent in patient simulations; for instance, emotional response to the situation, organizational factors, decisions made by physicians and societal conventions.

Another way to approach decision-making is by considering aspects of responsibility and 'locus of control'. Miller (1980) has shown that control is not always preferable to non-control in decision-making. Control is to be preferred only if the subject perceives that her/his actions will yield the desired result with certainty. In this study, the receptionist nurses were shown to face complex medical dilemmas during the telephone consultations. Hence, responsibility and independence should not be seen abstracted in isolation, but should be seen also from the point of view of the individual nurse in the work situation. Miller (1985) argues that the most important thing is what nurses are doing, not what they ought to do. Consequently, an increase in their medical responsibility should be accompanied by support measures, in terms of training, as well as concrete support in their daily work. Concerning training, the term 'nurse practitioner' has been used for a nurse with extra training who works with a large degree of autonomy in general practice (Stilwell *et al.*, 1987). Marklund *et al.* (1989) have developed a special educational programme for receptionist nurses with practical experience. This programme proved to increase both confidence and satisfaction with work among the participating nurses.

## Social dilemmas

Computerization is one solution that has been tried to solve the most prevalent organizational dilemma observed in this study: administration of the medical record. However, even though several attempts have been made, most computer-based medical record systems have been experimental in character, and have remained at the sites where they were developed. An exception is the COSTAR system, or versions thereof, which has been distributed internationally (Barnett, 1984). The main shortcomings of the computer-based record systems have been, in addition to costs, the human-computer interface and a resulting more rigid organization of work (Lind *et al.*, 1988). An alternative solution, which would benefit nurses, would be to computerize the administration of the medical record, and not the record as such, since the localization of the record is often the major problem.

Dilemmas in the communication with the patient occurred in one consultation out of three. In contrast to previous studies on physician–patient communication (Arborelius & Timpka, 1990; Plaja & Cohen, 1968; West, 1984), none of these dilemmas were of the type where the nurse had difficulty understanding the patient. This may be because the nurse's and patient's 'frames of reference' are more similar than those of the physician and patient.

The most common type of communication dilemma that the nurse faced was distrust, i.e. she felt that the patient did not speak entirely truthfully. Timpka & Arborelius (1990) also found that, for GPs, distrusting the patient was the most common communication dilemma. Millman (1977) has reported on patients distrusting care providers, and identified two major strategies by which physicians cope with perceived patient distrust: avoidance of the topic, and 'neutralization', i.e. the topic was redefined, and met with direct reassurance. Here, in the opposite situation, where the nurse distrusted the patient, the corresponding pattern was observed. The distrust very seldom became explicit in the conversation. Hence, questions like 'Do you really mean that?' were very uncommon.

One important issue challenging the nurses' personal competence concerned the settlement of the emotional distance between the nurse and patient. Llewelyn (1984) contends that closing down the emotional distance by deviating from the 'medical model', i.e. from emotional neutrality, is associated with a risk of emotional stress for the nurse. However, taking the risk may lead to personal growth if the emotional distance is settled at the right level for both the nurse and the patient. Since this level seems to be unique for every consultation, it also has to be dynamically settled for each consultation. This competence regarding settlement of emotional distance can only be learned by practice and feedback on the individual consultation style. There is a well-established consensus that such training or support is essential in nursing (e.g. Eastwood, 1985). On the other hand, the choice of methods for the training is still a matter of dispute (e.g. Fielding & Llewelyn, 1987). It is clear that training in the settlement of emotional distance cannot be provided as one-day or weekend 'self-discovery' courses. A possible form is a 'local support group', where recent emotionally stressful situations are discussed and from which organizational changes for support can be implemented directly.

For practice research, nursing has mainly relied on 'traditional' scientific methods (Moody *et al.*, 1989). Cull-Willby & Pepin (1987) point out that, in nursing, the practice of interpersonal interventions has been studied inadequately using methods designed to explain the physical world, but also that 'nursing is continuing to pursue new modes of inquiry'. Taylor-Myers & Haase (1989) contend that, for integration of qualitative and quantitative methods, both data sources should be considered equally important. This would guarantee the identification of issues where the participants' subjective views are different from the researchers' objectives. For this study, the solitary use of quantitative methods would have been especially inadequate, since dilemmas are situational and require detailed analyses.

The theory used for the classification structures in the study has similarities with epistemological theory suggested by Burnard (1987) as a basis for learning in nursing. Burnard's 'propositional' knowledge corresponds to the category 'medical–scientific knowledge' used here. However, Burnard's 'experiential' knowledge (i.e. personal knowledge gained through an encounter with a subject, person or thing) is, in the present classification structure, divided into social knowledge (i.e. knowledge of norms for social interaction) and personal competence (i.e. knowledge of one's own emotions and opinions, and their role in the interpretation of life events). Burnard's 'practical' knowledge has no correspondence in the present classification. Instead, all knowledge that is used in daily work is considered as practical and tacit 'knowhow' (see Benner, 1984). Only when a 'breakdown' in practice routines occurs (a dilemma) is reflection needed and knowledge becomes available at a cognitive level. Hence, in this view, practical knowledge is not available for explicit communication in a formal sense, and thus cannot be verbally reported.

### Action research

This study concerned description of the receptionist nurses' telephone consultations, and identification of the dilemmas that occurred. However, to bring about and evaluate the necessary changes, another type of process is necessary. The research findings have to be translated into the practice of receptionist nurses. In action research, the researcher is supposed to involve the group under study in acting upon research findings so that 'research becomes a resource that people can use to change their own lives' (Webb, 1989). Ketterer *et al.* (1980) describe five characteristics of action research:

(1) Collaboration between researchers and the action organization in terms of aims and performance of the research.
(2) Approval of the parallel goals of practical problem-solving and knowledge-building.
(3) Continuous feedback to participants of research findings, and also of results obtained by outside researchers.
(4) Recognition of group dynamics in the research process; attention is paid to values, power structure, opinion leaders, accepted experts, etc.
(5) Cyclical research process. Description, action and evaluation phases succeed each other in an uninterrupted cycle.

The findings of this investigation are, together with organizational studies (e.g. Timpka & Nyce, 1992), meant for use in processes aimed at changing and developing the work role of the receptionist nurse. Accordingly, the local continuation of this study is organized in an action research project where the researchers and nurses collaborate in a project group together with local health care administrators. The project has this far resulted in, amongst other things, a specially adapted information system (Timpka *et al.*, 1992).

## *References*

Arborelius, E. & Timpka, T. (1990) General practitioners comment on video-recorded consultations: what can we learn from these comments to understand the process in the patient–physician relationship. *Family Practice*, **7**, 84–90.

Barnett, G.O. (1984) The application of computer-based medical record systems in ambulatory practice. *New England Medical Journal*, **310**, 1643–50.

Benner, P. (1984) *From Novice to Expert.* Addison-Wesley, Menlo Park.

Bogdan, R. & Taylor, S.J. (1975) *Introduction to Qualitative Methods*, John Wiley, New York.

Burnard, P. (1987) Towards an epistemological basis for experiential learning in nurse education. *Journal of Advanced Nursing*, **12**, 189–93.

Cicourel, A.V. (1987) Cognitive and organizational aspects of medical diagnostic reasoning. *Discourse Processes*, **10**, 347–67.

Cull-Willby, B. & Pepin, J. (1987) Towards a co-existence of paradigms in nursing knowledge development. *Journal of Advanced Nursing*, **12**, 515–21.

de Graaf, E. (1989) A test of medical problem-solving scored by nurses and doctors: the handicap of expertise. *Medical Education*, **23**, 381–6.

Eastwood, C.M. (1985) The role of communication in nursing – perceptual variations in student/teacher responses in Northern Ireland. *Journal of Advanced Nursing*, **10**, 245–50.

Faulkner, A. (1979) Monitoring nurse–patient conversation in a ward. *Nursing Times*, **75**, 95–6.

Field, P.A. (1987) The impact of nursing theory on the clinical decision making process: *Journal of Advanced Nursing*, **12**, 563–71.

Fielding, R.G. & Llewelyn, B.A. (1987) Communication training in nursing may damage your health and enthusiasm: some warnings. *Journal of Advance Nursing*, **12**, 281–90.

Fisher, S. (1985) *Stress and Perception of Control.* Lawrence Erlbaum, London.

Habermas, J. (1979) What is Universal Pragmatics? In *Communication and the Evolution of Society*. Beacon Press, London.

Holtzemer, W.L. (1986) The structure of problem solving in simulations. *Nursing Research*, **35**, 231–6.

Kagan, C. (1985) *Interpersonal Skills in Nursing: Research and Applications*. Croom Helm, London.

Ketterer, R.F., Price, R.H. & Politser, E. (1980) The action research paradigm. In *Evaluation and Action in the Social Environment*. Academic Press, New York.

Lind, M., Petterson, E., Sandblad, B. & Schneider, W. (1988) Computer based workstations in health care. In *Towards New Hospital Information Systems* (eds A.R. Bakker, M.J. Ball, J.R. Sherrer & J.L. Willems, pp. 235–42. North Holland, Amsterdam.

Llewelyn, S.P. (1984) The cost of giving: emotional growth and emotional stress. In *Understanding Nurses* (ed. S. Skevington). John Wiley, Chichester.

Marklund, B. & Bengtsson, C. (1989) Medical advice by telephone at Swedish health centres: who calls and what are the problems. *Family Practice*, **6**, 42–6.

Marklund, B. Silfverhielm, B. & Bengtsson, C. (1989) Evaluation of an educational programme for telephone advisors in primary health care. *Family Practice*, **6**, 263–7.

Miller, A. (1985) The relationship between nursing theory and practice. *Journal of Advanced Nursing*, **10**, 417–24.

Miller, S.M. (1980) Why having control reduces stress: if I can stop the roller coaster, I don't want to get off. In *Human Helplessness. Theory and Applications*. (eds I. Garber & M.E.P. Seligman). Academic Press, New York.

Millman, M. (1977) *The Unkindest Cut*. Morrow, New York.

Moody, L.E., Wilson, M.E., Smyth, K., Schwartz, R., Tittle, M. & van Cott, M.L. (1989) Analysis of a decade of nursing practice research. *Nursing Research*, **37**, 374–9.

Morrison, P. & Burnard, P. (1989) Students' and trained nurses' perceptions of their own interpersonal skills: a report and comparison. *Journal of Advanced Nursing*, **14**, 321–9.

Newell, A. & Simon, H. (1973) *Human Problem Solving*. Prentice-Hall, New York.

Pendelton, D., Schofield, T., Tate, P. & Havelock, P. (1984) *The Consultation. An Approach to Learning and Teaching*. Oxford University Press, Oxford.

Plaja, A. & Cohen, S. (1968) Communication between physicians and patients in out-patient clinics: social and cultural factors. *Millbank Memorial Fund Quarterly*, **46**, 161–213.

Stilwell, B., Greenfield, S., Drury, V.W.M. & Hull, F.M. (1987) A nurse practitioner in general practice: working style and pattern of consultations. *Journal of the Royal College of General Practitioners*, **37**, 154–7.

Swedish Health and Medical Services Act SFS (1982): 763, SFS (1985): 560, Liber, Stockholm.

Tanner, C.A., Padrick, K.P., Westfall, U.E. & Putzier, D.J. (1987) Diagnostic reasoning strategies of nurses and nursing students. *Nursing Research*, **36**, 358–63.

Taylor-Myers, S. & Haase, J.E. (1989) Guidelines for integration of quantitative and qualitative approaches. *Nursing Research*, **38**, 299–301.

Timpka, T. & Arborelius, E. (1989) Study of the practitioner's knowledge need and use during health care consultations. Part 1: Theory and method. In *Proceedings of MedInfo '89* (eds B. Barber, C. Cao & G. Wagner). Elsevier, Amsterdam.

Timpka, T. & Arborelius, E. (1990) The GP's dilemmas: a study of knowledge need and use during health care consultations. *Methods of Information in Medicine*, **29**, 23–9.

Timpka, T. & Nyce, J.M. (1992) Dilemmas at a primary health care centre: a baseline study for computer supported health care work. *Methods of Information in Medicine*, **31**, 204–9.

Timpka, T., Nyce, J.M., Sjöberg, C. *et al* (1992) Developing a clinical hypermedia corpus: experiences from the use of a practice-centered method. In *Proceedings of SCAMC '92* (ed. M. Frisse), pp. 493–7. McGraw-Hill, New York.

Webb, C. (1989) Action research: philosophy, methods and personal experiences. *Journal of Advanced Nursing*, **14**, 403–10.

West, C. (1984) *Routine Complications. Troubles in Talk Between Doctors and Patients*. Indiana University Press, Bloomington.

Wilson-Barnett, J. (1988) Patient teaching or patient counselling? *Journal of Advanced Nursing*, **13**, 215–22.

Woods, N.F. (1984) Methods for studying diagnostic reasoning in nursing. In *Diagnostic Reasoning in Nursing* (ed. D.L. Carnevali). J.B. Lippincott, Philadelphia.

# Chapter 10
# Searching for health needs: the work of health visiting

KAREN I. CHALMERS, *RN, BScN, MSc (A), PhD*
Associate Professor, Faculty of Nursing, University of Manitoba, Winnipeg, Manitoba, Canada

Searching out health needs and stimulating clients' awareness of health needs are two key principles of British health visiting practice. However, there is little empirically based knowledge of how health visitors carry out these functions in their daily work. The purpose of this chapter is to describe and analyse health visitors' work in searching for health needs and promoting clients' awareness and actions in response to professionally identified needs. Forty-five health visitors were interviewed by means of semi-structured, conversational interviews. Findings identified that searching for health needs occurred in four types of situations. These were needs that were (a) client initiated, (b) easily seen, (c) 'opened up' by the health visitor, and (d) suspected and hidden. Several processes were involved in searching for needs and stimulating clients' awareness and actions, including: questioning, using illustrations from other client situations, normalizing, assigning homework, assessing and intervening while searching, and responding to cues. Timing played an important part in when and how interventions to search out needs occurred. This study contributes to our understanding of how health visitors work in the community to promote individual and family health.

## Introduction

Health visitors provide primary prevention services to individuals, families and groups in the community. An important component of this work involves searching out health needs and stimulating people's awareness of health needs. In the now classic document, *An Investigation into the Principles of Health Visiting* (Council for the Education and Training of Health Visitors, 1977), the importance of the identification and fulfilment of clients' self-declared and recognized, as well as unacknowledged and unrecognized, health needs, was outlined. Furthermore, the document emphasizes the importance of early detection of health needs in the first two principles of health visiting: (a) the search for health needs, and (b) the stimulation of the awareness of health needs.

Most of the literature on early detection and case finding addresses the importance of the health visitor's role in seeking out health needs and problems early (for example, Orr, 1985; Robertson, 1988). However, there has been little empirical investigation of the searching role in health visiting practice. Dobby (1986) attempted to develop a morbidity survey instrument to identify unmet needs in the under-five population. Other research has focused on screening postnatal mothers for depression (Briscoe, 1986; Hennessy, 1985). No empirical literature was identified which provides clarification of how health visitors conceptualize needs and the actual practice strategies used to search out needs. Indeed, the literature in general is lacking in empirical studies which capture the processes involved in health visiting practice.

## Little information

Much of the research on health visiting practice has used quantitative designs to measure health visitors' interventions to particular client groups (for example, studies reported in Clark's (1981) extensive review of the early health visiting research, and the more recent surveys such as While's (1985) epidemiological survey of health visiting services to young children), and quasi-experimental designs addressing the outcomes of health visitors' interventions (for example, Barker & Anderson, 1988; Carpenter, 1988; Colver & Pearson, 1985; Holden *et al.*, 1989). Despite the importance of these studies in describing health visitors' client groups and assessing the effectiveness of interventions, much of this research provides little information about what it is that health visitors do that contributes to positive outcomes.

Qualitative studies that address the processes in health visiting practice are increasingly seen as needed to enable more understanding of both the health visitor's and client's roles in the interaction processes and how these processes may influence client outcomes. Using interviews and observational methods, studies of health visitors' practice in child health clinics (Warner, 1984), during the primary (Montgomery-Robinson, 1987; Sefi, 1985) and other home visits (Clark, 1985; Cowley, 1991; Mason, 1988) have helped to make the processes of practice more visible.

## *The study*

No studies were found which described and analysed the case finding role in health visiting practice. Therefore, the purpose of this chapter is to contribute to further understanding of the processes involved in health visiting practice by describing and analysing health visitors' work in searching out and stimulating clients' awareness of health needs.

## *Method*

### Design

A qualitative design in a naturalist setting was employed in this study. Through the grounded theory approach (Glaser & Strauss, 1967; Strauss, 1987), health visitors' work in seeking out and promoting clients' awareness of needs was uncovered.

### Participants and settings

A convenience sample of 45 experienced health visitors based in 13 health authorities in the north-west of England participated in the study. Participants were experienced health visitors (mean = 10 years, range = 3.5–30 years), female, and primarily middle-aged. Both physician-attached and geographic work assignments, and generic and speciality programmes were represented by the health visitors in the sample. Participants were interviewed in their work sites ($n = 35$) or other convenient sites of their choosing ($n = 5$). The wide range of practice settings and practice experiences allowed for maximum variation in the data (Patton, 1980).

### Data collection

The grounded theory approach to data collection and analysis was used (Glaser & Strauss, 1967; Strauss, 1987; Strauss & Corbin, 1990). Data were collected by tape-recorded, conversational interviews (Lofland, 1976; Schatzman & Strauss, 1973), field notes on contextual factors which might influence the data collection process and product, and a short self-administered data sheet documenting socio-demographic and employment characteristics.

The interviews were organized around cases in which health visitors considered their interventions had a positive impact and cases in which their interventions had little impact. Most participants were interviewed alone ($n = 36$); three two-person and one three-person interviews were also conducted. According to the grounded theory tradition, the number of participants was not fixed prior to data collection. Data collection was deemed complete when no new information was forthcoming, all categories saturated, and the core category identified. Categories were not preconceived prior to the research project; as the analysis proceeded, key categories emerged and these were focused upon with other respondents in subsequent interviews.

*Analysis*

Analysis proceeded through the stages of open coding, building and saturating categories, and finally the identification of the core category (Charmaz, 1983; Glaser & Strauss, 1967; Glaser, 1978; Strauss, 1987). Constant comparison of data was used throughout the analysis (Charmaz, 1983; Strauss, 1987). Through the activities of theoretical sampling, category building, writing memos and diagramming (Corbin, 1986), the core category capturing the main psychosocial process in the data was identified (Strauss & Corbin, 1990). This formed the basis of the mid-range substantive process theory, labelled 'giving' and 'receiving' in health visiting practice.

In summary, the theory provided an explanation and understanding of how health visitors and clients interact. Both parties attempt to control the interactions by selectively making and receiving offers. What gets offered and received was a complex process related to the individual health visitors and clients, and the context in which the interactions took place. Health visitors' work of searching out health needs and stimulating clients' awareness of their health needs was a key category contributing to the process theory.

Throughout the study, measures were undertaken to enhance the rigour of the research process and hence the credibility of the research product. These procedures focused on measures to increase the credibility, fittingness, auditability and confirmability of the research findings (Brink, 1989; Glaser & Strauss, 1965; Glaser & Strauss, 1967; Lincoln & Guba, 1985; Sandelowski, 1986; Schatzman & Strauss, 1973). For a detailed outline of the process theory and the method used in the research, the reader is directed to previous published papers (Chalmers & Luker, 1991; Chalmers, 1992a,b).

## Findings: searching out and promoting awareness of health needs

### Types of situations

The work of searching out and promoting an awareness of health needs was a significant part of health visiting work. This work occurred in four types of situations: needs were initiated by the client; easily seen by the health visitor; 'opened up' by the health visitor; and suspected but hidden. Each is described briefly below.

*Client initiated*

In the first type of situation, clients identified needs or problems and sought out the health visitor or took the initiative and raised their concerns during a scheduled home visit. This category also included the identification of needs through routine screening procedures such as developmental assessments, hearing screenings, and breast screening clinics.

In these situations the client initiated action in response to an actual or potential need or problem and sought out the service or raised the concern with the health visitor. In client-initiated work, the health visitor's role may have involved widening the client's understanding of the need as part of the processes involved in assessing the situation and intervening. However, the work involved in stimulating the client's awareness of the need was not necessary.

*Easily seen*

In the second type of situation, the health visitor identified an easily observable need or problem during contact with the client. In these situations, the health visitor did not have to 'work' to uncover the need or problem. It was readily apparent to her. However, considerable work may have been involved in attempting to help the client see the presence of the need or problem.

These situations often involved physical health problems that were immediately apparent when the health visitor met the client. For example, one health visitor initiated contact with a family with three young children. She was new to the visiting area which had been under visited for some time. On her initial contact she discovered two of the children to be seriously ill and immediately initiated medical intervention. The children were subsequently admitted to hospital and found to have tuberculosis. In this example, the parents had not been aware of the severity of their children's illnesses. After discharge, the health visitor's interventions involved increasing the parents' awareness of health needs by helping them learn to recognize the signs of early illness in their children and to take appropriate action.

*'Opening up' the need*

In the third type of situation, the need or problem is uncovered during the course of the contact/visit through the process of 'opening up' the need or problem with the client. In these situations the need/problem may not have been immediately observable to the health visitor but later was uncovered during the course of the health visitor–client interactions. Considerable work was often involved in exploring the client situation in order to uncover and 'open up' the need or problem.

*Suspected hidden need*

In the final type of situation, the health visitor is concerned about a client; she suspects there is an unmet need or problem but is unable to 'open it up' and identify it. The health visitor's attempts to bring the health need 'out into the open' may be blocked by the client, or the health visitor may be unable to open up the need or problems because she has not learned how to do this. The health visitor identifies behaviours that show her that something in the client situation is 'not quite right', but she is unable to act on this.

**Processes involved in searching for and promoting clients' awareness of health needs**

Several factors influenced the processes in identifying needs and problems. These factors were related to the client, the health visitor, and the particular context in which the health visitor and client interacted. Each was interconnected and interrelated.

In order for a health need or problem to be sought out and identified, the health visitor must have a conceptualization of what it is she is looking for. When the health need is severe and readily observable, such as the example of the seriously ill children cited above, the search process was straightforward. However, in most of the situations discussed in the interviews, this process was far more complex. Health visitors used several processes to search out needs and stimulate clients' awareness of these needs. Each is discussed below.

*Questioning*

Health visitors used questioning to explore client situations and gather information. Questioning was commonly used when the health visitor had little information about the client situation; that is, in the traditional way to gather data. But questioning was also used to help clients explore and understand their situation more fully. For example, one health visitor used questioning as an intervention to help new mothers explore their reactions to first-time parenthood:

HV  'I think what I highlight a lot, especially with first mums, is how difficult they do find their roles as first parents. How they didn't expect to find it as difficult and responsible as they find it. I always bring that up by saying "How are you finding parenthood? It's quite difficult, isn't it, with a new baby here all the time?"'

In this situation the health visitor was not using questioning just to gather information about how the mother was adjusting to her new role, but was using questioning also as an intervention to help the client examine her situation.

   In other situations, questioning was used to 'open up' needs or problems which the health visitor was aware of or suspected may be present. Questioning may allow topics to be opened up which the client may be unable to initiate independently. For example, one health visitor had been visiting a new mother whose baby experienced asphyxia at birth. At this point the hospital was uncertain about the permanent damage to the baby and communicated little information to the parents. The health visitor discussed how she attempted to pace herself with the mother's need for information by the use of skilful questioning:

HV   'I think it's always a problem as to when you broach the subject [of handicap]. I initially said, "Are you happy with the care you're getting from the hospital?" and she started crying then. Because he'd [baby] been in the hospital recently with a viral infection and had been sick and poorly. She felt she had been given no time at all. Following that, which had upset her quite a bit, I asked her whether she was happy with things at the physio, doctors, developmental doctor, etc., and I think I asked her then whether anyone had discussed with her what David's condition could be.'

By exploring the mother's satisfaction with her child's care, this health visitor was able to open up a discussion of the handicap at a time when the mother appeared to want information. Through this process, she was able to provide information and support and later to initiate interventions with the hospital to provide this mother with more support and information. Questioning in this example helped identify a need and led to interventions to help meet the need. Questioning as an intervention has the potential to enable health visitors to seek out needs, but also can be used to assist clients to become more fully aware of their needs.

*Using illustrations from other client situations*

Illustrations from their work with other clients can also be used to help health visitors open up needs or problems which they identify or suspect are present in clients. In this way the clients can relate to a concrete example when disclosing a similar need. For example, one health visitor described to the researcher (R) how she uncovered relationship problems a young couple was having after the birth of their first child:

HV   'I brought up problems that I could see would happen and she agreed to these. I had to draw it out by giving illustrations. She couldn't come out with them and say, "I'm having problems with him. I'm not sleeping with him and he wants to sleep with me and I can't."
R     How would you say this?

HV    I found over the years, I use illustrations from other families I've met. I would say something like, "Some families with a new baby find problems with this or that" and then she would say she was having a problem too ... She would identify with what I've said.'

By using concrete examples from other client situations, the health visitor was able to help the client become aware of similar needs in her own situation. The client was then receptive to interventions to help address these needs.

*Normalizing*

Another approach health visitors used to explore potential needs and help clients acknowledge them was to normalize the occurrence of needs or problems. By acknowledging specific needs or problems as part of the usual experiences in living, health visitors attempted to create an environment for disclosure and effective collaborative intervention.

For example, a health visitor explored the mother–daughter relationship by normalizing relationship conflicts that occur between parents and children. In this example, the mother had sought out the health visitor for help with enuresis in her school-aged daughter.

HV    'I find that if you're talking, the questions that you ask allow the flood gates to open. You don't have to drag it out of them. With many of them, something has been there for a very long time that's never been voiced and you've only got to ask the right question and it all floods out. It's a case of saying, "How do you and Gwen get on together? Do you have disagreements like most parents and children do? Do you find that she's a pain sometimes?" And mum saying, "I really can't handle her, she drives me potty."

R    It sounds like you give her permission to say that?

HV    Yes, you've got to put it to them that the way they're feeling is sometimes quite normal.'

This health visitor went on to discuss how she sometimes used self-disclosure to normalize that all parents find their children problematic at times:

HV    'I would say to some of my mums, "My son drives me mad. He's got school phobia; every morning it's a battle to get him to school ... there are days when I could throw him out of the window" or I say "Go away. I've had enough of you." They click on to that and say that they feel like that too sometimes. You've got to have some sort of situation where it's acceptable to say that.'

By normalizing many common feelings, and at times disclosing their own, health visitors attempted to create a climate in which needs could be disclosed.

*Assigning homework*

Another process to assist clients to become more aware of their particular health needs and their motivation to change was to give them some type of homework assignment. This approach was only seen as effective in highly motivated clients. In the following example, a woman sought out the health visitor with concerns about her pre-school child's refusal to sleep in his own bed:

HV    '... she described the problem and I suggested, to get a clearer view of the problem, to write it down, exactly what the child's behaviour was over one week, to write down exactly what was happening ... it would give us something to latch on to, and I could go back and we could talk things over ... I had suggested the diary because I think, for one thing, it shows how motivated they are. I didn't say that to them [both parents were present for the interview] but I mean, if they've done it, it would also give them something practical to do. Also, it shows you how seriously they view the problem, how much effort they are prepared to put in.'

*Assessing and intervening while searching*

Although health visitors searched for needs through many of the processes described above, often multiple processes occurred at the same time. A common example was the 'search within a search'. While the health visitor was searching out one health need, she frequently was assessing other potential needs and intervening to promote health at the same time. For example, a health visitor assessed the speech of a two-year-old child whom the mother had concerns about not speaking. At the same time she was assessing the mother–child interaction and role modelling interaction patterns for the mother. The screening of the speech was just one assessment intervention while searching for and stimulating the awareness of other needs.

*Responding to cues*

In many situations the health concern was not immediately apparent or was not unearthed through the processes of exploring and questioning. Health visitors frequently were alert to cues in situations which later enabled them to move closer to opening up needs and problems. Being alert to cues that a need or a problem existed was an important component of the search process. Health visitors used their previous professional experiences and their own life experiences to cue them that something in the situation was 'not quite right'. The term 'cue' in these situations referred to 'a sign or intimation when to speak or act; a hint' (*Shorter Oxford English Dictionary*, 1980).

Learning to be alert to cues and responding to cued information was an important part of searching out health needs. Health visitors who could effectively recognize and act on cues could move beyond the presenting health needs and problems to uncover unrecognized or unacknowledged health needs. The following illustrations from the data provide examples of how being alert to cues and responding to them assisted in identifying health needs.

In one situation, a health visitor uses her experience from other similar cases as a backdrop to identify that something in a family situation was 'not quite right'. In this case, the woman was somewhat depressed after the birth of her baby:

HV   'The [client's] mother never baby-sat, although she lived nearby. For a grandmother and the first grandchild, I thought that was strange ... She frequently said that she had more confidence in me, that I had more or less replaced her mother, that she would talk to me. So she used me as a confidant to a certain extent.'

This health visitor compared this situation with others from her past experiences and noted that the grandmother's behaviour was atypical. While this behaviour in itself was not conclusive of an unmet health need, the absence of typical 'grandmothering' behaviour cued this health visitor to pay close attention to the level of support that this woman was receiving. This situation later resulted in the woman disclosing familial childhood incest of which the client claimed her mother was aware.

In another example, the health visitor was not able to identify what in the situation was 'not quite right'. In this situation, a baby with a cleft palate was having a great deal of difficulty retaining feeds. The hospital staff were not able to find anything wrong with the baby and were labelling the problems as an 'anxious mother':

HV   'Although the hospital had put it down to being an anxious mother, I felt that there was something else because I'd just never had that problem feeding a cleft palate baby myself, but I couldn't put my finger on it and everyone was coming up with, you know, "she's putting her anxieties on the baby", but she [mother] also thought there was something else wrong, and I think mothers normally know ... it just wasn't right, and while I would take into account what everyone else was saying, it still didn't seem quite right...'

The health visitor was responding to some cues in the situation that she, herself, was not quite knowledgeable of. These cues appeared to keep her focused on other possible explanations for the baby's problems and when she subsequently saw the baby vomit, she considered the likely cause of the feeding problem to be a food allergy. The baby was subsequently medically diagnosed and thrived on a soya formula.

Cues can alert the health visitor to factors in the situation with clients that are 'not quite right'. In other situations, cues were used to identify that the client was proceeding along a 'normal' course. In one example, a health visitor used cues to assess a mother's mood after the birth of the second child. After her first baby, the woman had sustained a very severe postnatal depression requiring hospitalization. The health visitor was able to sort out the cues she was attending to in order to ascertain that, in this situation, the woman's emotional response was within the usual range of postnatal adjustment:

HV  'I think if she had been very tearful or very withdrawn [I would have been concerned]. She was always able to say how she felt ... and she really did so well and was super with the baby and breast fed beautifully...'

The health visitor assessed the cues in this situation and concluded that the mother's anxiety and fatigue were within the usual responses.

### Difficulty in articulating
Health visitors were not always able to articulate easily what cues in situations they were actually responding to. Sometimes health visitors had difficulty articulating what cues they were responding to that enabled them to assess that a situation was likely to be all right or potentially problematic. When pressed, though, they were sometimes able to identify what criteria in the situation they were using for their assessment. It appeared as if some criteria were buried within their experiences of many similar cases and were not immediately available for discussion.

For some health visitors these cues were part of an almost undercover assessment producing a kind of 'sixth sense' in their work. For example, one health visitor worked with a young woman who had two small children and was pregnant with twins. Despite this woman's very troubled background and explosive behaviour, the health visitor felt fairly confident that she would not abuse her children:

HV  'I think everything is always a gut feeling, really, because you never really know. I mean it's a big responsibility to say, "I don't think that these children will come to any harm" ... but at some point you've got to look at it and say, "you know, well, no I don't think so, I feel confident."

R    Can you think back, what was in the situation that allowed you to feel confident about that...?

HV    Well she could, you know, it was possible she could blow her top on them and that, you know, things like that have happened. It's just that sometimes, you know, that situation is just right for that ... and well I think because of the husband really ... even though he's an unstable character in lots of ways, as far as job wise is concerned, I think over the years that they are closer. The relationship is much better and that he seems to be doing more for her, you know.'

Despite difficulty in articulating what criteria she was using to assess this situation, the health visitor was attending to cues that the mother was basically able to cope with the children.

In addition to using cues in the clients' present or recent past situation to alert them to areas to explore in the present, health visitors used events from the clients' childhood to alert them to possible current health needs. Past events, such as the death of parents, difficult childhoods and care placements, and other problems provided cues to assess current functioning more carefully.

The following example outlines how a health visitor used the information that a young woman's parents were killed when she was a young teenager to assess her current parenting more fully. The mother had been giving the baby Ribena (blackcurrant drink) in a bottle and the baby had severely decayed teeth:

HV    'This mother didn't know how to calm the child. She was obviously very anxious if her little baby cried. She hadn't got her own mother to educate her, so I had to show her how to be a mother.'

By using her background knowledge of the mother's past, the health visitor assessed the dental problem within a broader framework and developed interventions to deal with health needs beyond the dental caries:

HV    'We were going through diet, child management, going through teenage years, going through the grieving process, making her grow to be an adult ... I tried to make her strong enough so that when the baby cried she would have the confidence to say, "You don't need anything now, you've just been fed" and go for a walk or something.'

The health visitor used her knowledge of the past to view the needs of this client more broadly.

**Timing**

Cues were helpful to alert the health visitor to situations that needed more careful assessment with the goal that problems might be unearthed and effective interventions put into place. The timing, though, was crucial in many situations. To get the timing wrong might jeopardize any effective work with some clients. Cues may alert the health visitor to a potential need or problem but the health visitor may not work at opening up the need at that particular time.

Health visitors often suspected that there were unmet needs but clients were not always ready to pursue the issue when the health visitor attempted to open up the problem or need. By noting the cues, though, the health visitor could be alert to opportunities to pursue the health issue at a later time. For example, one health visitor described her attempts to provide services for a single career woman in her thirties with a new baby. This woman was new to the community and had few supports. The health visitor had attempted to explore the woman's coping abilities and possible need for external supports earlier but the woman was resistant to services except clinic services:

HV  'I was thinking that something was very wrong here [the woman had exploded in clinic when she had been called by the wrong name] as I would have suspected from the first visit ... I had done a couple of follow-up visits after she had first come here but I had rather a block. Gone so far offering help and exploring areas with her and then I felt I was intruding and I think you shouldn't go on if the client doesn't want to say anything at the time. So I left it with her to contact me.'

Although noting that there were areas of likely concern, the health visitor was not able to get the problems 'opened up'. Later, after the woman's emotional outburst in clinic, the health visitor used the opportunity of the one-year-old visit to contact the woman again. At this point, she was able to 'open up' a discussion of the woman's coping with single parenting and collaboratively initiate services to decrease her isolation. The timing of the exploration of problems appeared critical to helping this woman meet her needs.

The timing has to be right before many needs and problems can be successfully opened up and dealt with. To move too quickly with some clients may result in them withdrawing further and denying the presence of health needs. The context in which health visitors work is also important and influences how timing is used. Since many clients, particularly families with young children, have not asked for home visiting services, they may not be wanting some needs or problems dealt with at the time that they are noted or suspected by the health visitor. To try to move too quickly may result in withdrawal of the client and, possibly even difficulty in gaining access.

*Could not wait*

Despite the importance accorded to getting the timing right when attempting to open up needs and problems, health visitors sometimes felt that they could not wait for a better time, that they had to act. The antecedents of these situations were actual or potential threats to the immediate health of family members, particularly children. For example, in one situation the health visitor had concerns about the household environment in a family with two children under two years. The house was cold, damp and dirty. In this case the health needs were clearly observable to the health visitor, but the processes to stimulate an awareness of the needs were much more complex. The health visitor had attempted to open up discussion of the environment without offending the parents; however, this had brought about no changes. Finally, with the advent of cold weather, she considered that she must act:

> HV   'We were getting to the time of year when I couldn't really delay because of the danger of cold injury to the baby. I think I got to the point where I went on this visit and the hands were swollen and I had to come on very strong on that visit and [said] "But whatever else you do, I know you don't feel like keeping the house clean and nice" which is the same as saying, "It's filthy" but put in a different way, isn't it, but you must keep your child warm ... I mean his hands were red and slightly swollen and, you know, they thought he'd got some infection and I said, "I think it's the cold" ...'

The arrival of the cold weather provided the impetus for the health visitor to act and confront the parents about the impact of their household environment on the children.

Waiting for the right time before attempting to open up needs or stimulate an awareness of needs in clients did not always result in getting the need or problem attended to. Sometimes the right timing never seemed to come. When health visitors had concerns about the well-being of clients, particularly children, they often had to forego waiting until the time seemed opportune to initiate action. Health visitors' work in these and other difficult situations is described elsewhere (Chalmers, 1992c).

## Constructing needs

The previous discussion had focused on the types of search situations and the processes involved in searching out and stimulating an awareness of health needs. These processes, though, did not occur in isolation. Health visitors' selective attention to some needs and not others was constructed within the social world of health visiting practice. Several factors influenced the search for some needs and the bypassing of other needs.

The availability of resources to assist with needs was a key factor which influenced health visitors' search for needs and stimulation of awareness of needs in clients. When follow-up or referral sources were not available, health visitors often hesitated to explore health issues with clients. Opening up a need when there were no referral agents or time for the health visitor herself to pursue the problem left the client with an acknowledged problem but with no help.

For example, one health visitor discussed her hesitation to explore with clients their motivation to stop smoking because of the lack of resources in the community and her own lack of time to initiate a stop-smoking programme:

HV   'I sometimes maybe see the need and I have to forget about it because I haven't got the time to pursue it. I can give one example at the hypertension clinic ... I ask them something related to smoking because it is pertinent to high blood pressure and heart disease, but I am frightened of asking if they want to give it up. I advise them that they should give up smoking but I am frightened of saying "Would you like some help to give up" because basically I haven't got the time. Because I know in my mind the best way to help someone to give up smoking is to do it in group therapy. I realize that ... but I haven't got an hour each week or whatever it is ... [Also] the clientele that I am dealing with is, I have to give them the motivation as well. I could do that. And I've got to retain the service for them fairly locally, I think, for it to be effective. I could do it ...'

This health visitor had assessed the need and the prerequisites to meet the need, but was unable to see that she could address the need within her existing time resources.

In the above example, the health visitor's hesitation to search out and stimulate an awareness of health needs connected with smoking was related to the concern of the time involved in starting up a new service for clients. Health visitors also made decisions about allocating time within their existing services. The most common decisions were related to how much time a particular client or family, with multiple needs, should be allocated. This decision was based on criteria largely within the health visitor's own conceptualization of her practice.

Health visitors appeared to operate according to their own frameworks for practice which guided how they allocated their time resources within their existing caseload. When they perceived that there was a need which fitted with their own conceptualization of need, they often went to great lengths to attempt to meet the need. For example, some health visitors gave out their home telephone numbers and encouraged clients to call them after clinic hours; they made home visits during evenings and on weekends; one brought

Christmas dinner to an elderly housebound person, and another even helped
a client paint her flat.

In the following example, a health visitor analysed her decision to provide
a young single woman with almost unlimited time and support over a four-
year period:

HV  'A lot of our work takes a lot of time and you don't often know which
way it will go. You have to balance it against the others and the
amount of input into it.
R    Did you have a hunch that this girl could "make it"?
HV  Yes, I did. I think I said earlier on, because when I stopped and thought
about it, "Am I doing the right thing here?" and balanced how much
input I'm putting into one family, I had a strong feeling it was right for
this family... There just seemed to be something about this girl that
made me feel, maybe the experience, all these things that we pull
together, that she wanted desperately to be a "good mother" and that
it was very important for her to be a good mother and that she had it in
her to be a good mother, given the right set of circumstances ...'

*Investment of time*

In this situation the health visitor invested considerable time in this young
woman to assist her to manage her own life and to parent more effectively. In
examining factors which influenced this considerable time and energy
investment, it appeared that the woman's response to the health visitor and
the health visitor's conceptualization of the client's situation were key factors
in the health visitor's long-term commitment to this client. The woman, and
her partner prior to the termination of their relationship, would initiate
contact with the health visitor with concerns about the baby. The woman
responded to the health visitor's advice for child care by initiating the
recommended practices. Her positive response to the health visitor enabled
many needs to be unearthed and additional help to be mobilized. It can be
seen that the client received the health visitor's offer and responded by giving
back to the health visitor.

Also, there were factors in the situation that appeared to have a positive
appeal to the health visitor. The client was perceived as trying very hard to
cope despite a difficult background (her mother had deserted her as a young
child), a postnatal depression, and a partner who was unsupportive and
critical of her mothering. After the partner's return to prison, and when the
child was a little older, the woman found part-time work to help support
herself and the child. These factors, the client's responsiveness to the health
visitor and her efforts to parent effectively and to become self-sufficient,
appeared to influence the health visitor and keep her fully engaged with the

client and her needs. The behaviours that the client was demonstrating appeared to 'fit' with the values of this health visitor: her conceptualization of a client fully worthy of her time and commitment. Thus, the health visitor attempted to address this client's needs to the upper limits of her knowledge and resources.

*No response from clients*

A different pattern occurred when clients did not respond or give back to their health visitors. In situations in which clients did not respond to health visitors, the pattern of staying fully committed in order to search out the health needs and help clients meet the needs was less evident. In families with young children health visitors did not 'desert' clients – they continued to visit – but adhered to the more routine component of their work, focusing primarily on child surveillance activities.

This pattern of focusing on the routine was particularly evident when clients needed material or service resources that were not readily available in the community and did not perceive the health visitor's 'offers' of support as helpful. When clients did not respond by receiving the offer of support and by opening up to the health visitor with other concerns, the health visitor is left in a difficult position. She may suspect that there are other needs in the family (some of which she may be able to help with, either by herself or by referring) but she is unable to get at the needs. By not being able to give help which is perceived as helpful by the client, both health visitor and client experience discomfort in their interactions. The usual consequence of an unsatisfactory interaction was for both parties to withdraw either partially or fully from the interactions.

In the following example, the health visitor was unable to help with housing problems and nursery placements for a family with four young children. She suspected that there were other problems in the family but was unable to get at the needs:

HV 'It was one of those situations where she [mother] was very mono-syllabic. I felt uncomfortable because I felt that they didn't really see that I was there for any particular reason. ... I suppose her negative response made me not particularly inclined to try. I know there are more things I could have done to try to build up the relationship but I didn't out of pure discouragement really. I felt there were not a lot of practical things that could be done – housing problem, finding a nursery placement for the child. When you feel there's really nothing you can do because there's very little you can do with the housing problems, you feel, "Why am I going?" and "What can she see that I've got to offer?" She wasn't a very open person so it wasn't as if she would find even talking about problems [helpful]. She wouldn't communicate by nature . . .'

This client's lack of response influenced the health visitor. She made fewer visits and gradually 'tried' less hard to open up problems. The client was not without services (she continued to receive clinic services for the children), but received less of the health visitor's efforts to get at other needs that she suspected were present in the family.

### Discussion

An important part of health visitors' work as uncovered in this study was searching out needs and attempting to stimulate clients' awareness of needs. However, health visitors do not offer all clients the same level of service and the same amount of their time and interest. The construction of what is considered a need or problem worthy of the health visitor's attention and action was influenced by many factors. With the exception of overt and serious physical health problems, construction of need was influenced by the health visitor's previous and current interactions in the social world. Health visitors responded positively to clients who received their offers of service by opening up with information and by acting on health visiting advice. They also appeared to be influenced by their conceptualization of the overall social worth of the client situation. While not refusing service, particularly in families with young children, they selectively 'gave' their offers of time and commitment.

Selective attention to patients is not a new finding. The influence of practitioners' assessment of the social worth of clients has been noted in many previous studies (Glaser & Strauss, 1965; Schwartz, 1975; Sudnow, 1967). Roth (1986) considered that all clients are 'evaluated' by health care staff in two ways: their worthiness for service (their social worth) and their legitimacy, that is their appropriateness to the professionals' concept of their work.

Based on his study of hospital emergency room services, Roth (1986) surmised that these two concepts are likely to be in operation in any professional service and to influence how services are dispensed. In this study of health visitors, it also appeared that some clients met health visitors' conceptualization of clients as fully worthy of the extra time, effort or services often required to search out and respond to needs. However, clients' social worth was not the only factor influencing their conceptualization; clients' responsiveness to health visitors' offers was also a critical factor. When clients were conceptualized as 'worthy' and responded positively to health visitors' efforts, health visitors often made efforts 'beyond the call of duty' to search out needs and provide assistance.

### Conceptualization and interpersonal skills

Many needs that health visitors identified were uncovered through the process of 'opening up' needs and problems as they interacted with clients. In order for this to occur, though, health visitors must have a conceptualization of what potential needs may be present in particular client situations and have the interpersonal skills to interview effectively to get at the needs. They also require the judgement to know when pursuing a potential need or problem would be detrimental for the client at that particular time. Judgement in knowing how and when to open up needs and problems that clients are not acknowledging and when and how to stimulate clients to make changes in their lives were skills that many health visitors in this study had learned and practised in their day-to-day work. Health visitors, however, receive little assistance in developing and enhancing their interpersonal skills.

Research into health visitor training reveals that knowledge of a technical and scientific nature is highly valued and taught to students (Twinn, 1990, personal communication). However, little attention is paid to the theoretical basis for the processes of assessing interpersonal competence in training. This is not surprising since the interpersonal component of health visiting has received little systematic study to date. Empirical research on American hospital nurses is uncovering the knowledge that is embedded in experienced practitioners (Benner, 1984; Benner & Tanner, 1987; Benner & Wrubel, 1989). Much more work is needed in health visiting to uncover how interpersonal skills are learned and used to open up needs and problems in clients and to stimulate clients' awareness of these needs.

Another factor which may influence health visitors' searching and stimulating intervention is their knowledge of and comfort with their own personal life issues. Health visitors may resist exploring and opening up problems that they are uncomfortable in dealing with, such as sexual abuse of children. Health visitors, like all professionals, need time and opportunities to explore their feelings related to their own and client life experiences in order to become more comfortable in working in these stressful situations. If professionals continue to practise without these issues resolved, they may miss many opportunities to help clients identify problems and seek out solutions.

The issue of searching out problems also presents ethical dilemmas. Health visitors were often aware of actual or potential client problems but were hesitant to explore health issues in more depth when they had no referral resources to offer clients or when they themselves were too busy to provide additional services. Health visitors seldom took this information and used it to pressure their health authority to develop services to address the identified needs. Their practice with individuals and families seemed to keep them focused at the micro level of practice, even when changes in the wider community were obviously necessary to address needs.

### Emphasis on child health

Several factors also influence which needs were searched for in health visiting practice. Searching for health needs occurred in the midst of a predominant focus on families with young children. The emphasis on child health in the health visiting service was a key factor affecting the time available to search for needs in both the young families and in other populations. The continual referral of new babies in the health visitor's caseload and the frequent 'routine' visiting of infants and young children provided both an opportunity and a restraint to searching for needs.

Caseloads often were driven by the influx of new babies. When the birth rate in the health visitor's caseload was high, her other work was not attended to as much. Conversely, when the birth rate falls, other work which could be attended to often was not started because of concerns that the birth rate may rise again. This lack of control of the flow of new baby 'work' into the health visitor's caseload affected health visitors' commitment to other kinds of work that might result in finding unmet needs.

Health visitors have demonstrated positive outcomes in working with other client groups such as elderly people in speciality programmes (Davies, 1990; Luker, 1982; Vetter *et al*, 1984; Victor & Vetter, 1985). However, work with this client group and others will not likely occur on a wide scale if the time for this work is not available.

The general practitioners' contracts arising from the British government's White Paper on primary health care (Department of Health and Social Security, 1987) may also have significant implications for health visitors' work in searching out needs. The employment of practice nurses and other health workers to carry out screening of patients may restrict the exploration of other needs and focus the client contacts solely on the body part or function being screened.

It was obvious from this study that many health visitors were able to uncover health concerns through their routine contact with clients. However, if health personnel do not have the necessary background knowledge to be cognizant of other health concerns that may be present, and the necessary skills to 'get at them', many opportunities to promote clients' health may be missed.

Anyone can be taught to carry out screening procedures, but the better prepared person is usually carrying out other assessments and interventions while screening. However, reducing the 'routine' work of health visiting may also have positive outcomes. Delegating 'routine' tasks to less well prepared workers may provide opportunities for health visitors to work with other client groups, such as elderly people, and to develop other approaches to their work.

## The future

Despite the importance of working with individuals and families to search out health needs, many clients' health needs will not be effectively met through interventions directed solely to individuals and families. Other approaches, such as community development initiatives and 'healthy public policies', are critical for health enhancement of populations (Ashton & Seymour, 1988; Downie *et al.*, 1990; Milio, 1986; Research Unit in Health and Behavioural Change, 1989). With increasing skill in working at the 'macro level', health visitors could use their knowledge of needs gained while working with individuals and families to have a wider impact on the community's health. In this way, the principle of searching out health needs and stimulating an awareness of health needs is addressed at the level of the community.

Current changes in the health care system in the UK, however, may limit the development of newer roles for health visitors. A recent study on staffing levels for community nurses (Social Policy Research Unit, 1993) documented many proposals for the delivery of community health services from purchases and providers of health services. The implementation of 'skills mix', the development of a 'generic' community nurse, and increased control by general practitioners over community nursing services will alter health visitors' practice in the community. Perhaps the most effective proposal comes from Barker (1993). He proposes that health visitors specialize as either essentially a practice or community health visitor. The practice health visitor would be responsible for all preventive and health promotion clinic work while the community specialist health visitor would take on regular home based work with high risk families and the wider community health promotion role.

Regardless of the model of community care which is eventually enacted, though, it is critical that re-alignment of health roles does not result in a reduction of primary and secondary preventive services in the community. Searching out health needs, stimulating an awareness of need, and addressing the needs will continue to be critical preventive functions.

## Acknowledgement

The author wishes to acknowledge and thank Professor Karen Luker for her advice on the research project from which this paper was developed. Dr Luker holds the Chair in Community Nursing at the University of Liverpool.

## References

Ashton, J. & Seymour, H. (1988) *The New Public Health.* Open University Press, Milton Keynes.

Barker, W. (1993) Patch and practice: specialist roles for health visitors. *Health Visitor*, **66**(6), 200–203.

Barker, W. & Anderson, R. (1988) *The Child Development Programme: An Evaluation of Process and Outcomes.* Evaluation Document 9. University of Bristol, Bristol.

Benner, P. & Tanner, C. (1987) How expert nurses use intuition. *American Journal of Nursing*, **87**, 23–31.

Benner, P. & Wrubel, J. (1989) *The primacy of caring: stress and coping in health and illness.* Addison-Wesley Co., Menlo Park, California.

Benner, P. (1984) *From Novice to Expert: Excellence and Power in Clinical Nursing Practice.* Addison-Wesley, London.

Brink, P. (1989) Issues in reliability and validity. In *Qualitative Nursing Research: A Contemporary Dialogue* (ed. J. Morse), pp. 151–68. Aspen Publications, Rockville, Maryland.

Briscoe, M. (1986) Identification of emotional problems in postpartum women by health visitors. *British Medical Journal*, **292**, 1245–8.

Carpenter, R. (1988) Preventing unexpected infant deaths by giving extra care to high risk infants. *Health Visitor*, **61**(8), 238–40.

Chalmers, K.I. (1992a) Working with men: an analysis of health visiting practice in families with young children. *International Journal of Nursing Studies*, **29**(1), 3–16.

Chalmers, K.I. (1992b) Giving and receiving: an empirically derived theory on health visiting practice. *Journal of Advanced Nursing*, **17**(11), 1317–25.

Chalmers, K.I. (1992c) Difficult work: health visitors' work with clients in the community. Unpublished paper. University of Manitoba, Winnipeg, Manitoba.

Chalmers, K.I. & Luker, K.A. (1991) The development of the health visitor– client relationship. *Scandinavian Journal of Caring Sciences*, **5**, 33–41.

Charmaz, K. (1983) The grounded theory method: an explication and interpretation. In *Contemporary Field Work* (ed. R. Emerson), pp. 109–26. Little, Brown, Boston.

Clark, J. (1981) *What Do Health Visitors Do? A Review of the Research 1960–1980.* Royal College of Nursing, London.

Clark, J. (1985) The process of health visiting. Unpublished PhD thesis. Polytechnic of the South Bank, London.

Colver, A. & Pearson, P. (1985) Safety in the home: how well are we doing? *Health Visitor*, **58**(2), 41–2.

Corbin, J. (1986) Qualitative data analysis for grounded theory. In *From Practice to Grounded Theory: Qualitative Research in Nursing* (W.C. Chenitz & J.M. Swanson), pp. 91–101. Addison-Wesley, Wokingham.

Council for the Education and Training of Health Visitors (1977) *An Investigation into the Principles of Health Visiting.* CETHV, London.

Cowley, S. (1991) A symbolic awareness context identified through a grounded theory study of health visiting. *Journal of Health Visiting*, **16**(6), 648–56.

Davies, S. (1990) An approach to case-finding the elderly. *Nursing Times*, **86**(51), 48–51.

Department of Health and Social Security (1987) *Promoting Better Health: The Government's Programme for Improving Primary Health Care.* HMSO, London.

Dobby, J. (1986) *The Development and Testing of a Method for Measuring the Need for and the Value of Routine Health Visiting.* The Health Promotion Research Trust, London.

Downie, R.S., Fyfe, C. & Tannahill, A. (1990) *Health Promotion: Models and Values.* Oxford University Press, Oxford.

Glaser, B. (1978) *Theoretical Sensitivity.* The Sociology Press, Mill Valley, California.

Glaser, B., & Strauss, A. (1965). The purpose and credibility of qualitative research. *Nursing Research*, **15**, 56–61.

Glaser, B. & Strauss, A. (1967) *The Discovery of Grounded Theory.* Aldine, Chicago.

Hennessy, D. (1985) Mothers and health visitors (abstract). Unpublished PhD thesis. University of Southampton, Southampton.

Holden, J., Sagovsky, R. & Cox, J. (1989) Counselling in a general practice setting: controlled study of health visitor intervention in treatment of postnatal depression. *British Journal of Medicine*, **298**, 223–226.

Lincoln, Y. & Guba, E. (1985) *Naturalistic Inquiry*. Sage, London.

Lofland, J. (1976) *Doing Social Life*. John Wiley, New York.

Luker, K.A. (1982) *Evaluating Health Visiting Practice: An Experimental Study to Evaluate the Effects of Focused Health Visitor Intervention on Elderly Women Living Alone at Home*. Royal College of Nursing, London.

Mason, C. (1988) Problems in health visiting: an anthropological study. Unpublished PhD thesis. Queen's University of Belfast, Belfast.

Milio, N. (1986) *Promoting Health Through Healthy Public Policy*. Canadian Public Health Association, Ottawa.

Montgomery-Robinson, K. (1987) The social construction of health visiting. Unpublished PhD thesis. The Polytechnic of the South Bank, London.

Orr, J. (1985) Assessing individual and family health needs in *Health Visiting* (eds. K. Luker & J. Orr), pp. 67–120. Blackwell Scientific Publications, Oxford.

Patton, M.Q. (1980) *Qualitative Evaluation Methods*. Sage, Beverly Hills, California.

Research Unit in Health and Behavioural Change, University of Edinburgh (1989) *Changing The Public Health*. John Wiley & Sons, Chichester.

Robertson, C. (1988) *Health Visiting in Practice*. Churchill Livingstone, Edinburgh.

Roth, J.A. (1986) Some contingencies of the moral evaluation and control of clientele: the case of hospital emergency service. In *The Sociology of Health and Illness: Critical Perspectives*, 2nd edn, (eds P. Conrad & R. Kern), pp. 322–33. St Martin's Press, New York.

Sandelowski, M. (1986) The problem of rigor in qualitative research. *Advances in Nursing Science*, **8**(3), 27–37.

Schatzman, L. & Strauss, A. (1973) *Field Research Strategies for a Natural Sociology*. Prentice-Hall, Englewood Cliffs, New Jersey.

Schwartz, B. (1975) *Queuing and Waiting: Studies in the Social Organization of Access and Delay*. University of Chicago Press, London.

Sefi, S. (1985) The first visit: a study of health visitor–mother verbal interaction. Unpublished master's dissertation. University of Warwick, Coventry.

*Shorter Oxford English Dictionary* (1980) Clarendon Press, Oxford.

Social Policy Research Unit (1993) *Nursing by Numbers? Setting Staffing Levels for District Nursing and Health Visiting Services*. University of York, York.

Strauss, A. & Corbin, J. (1990) *Basics of Qualitative Research: Grounded Theory Procedures and Techniques*. Sage, Newbury Park, California.

Sudnow, D. (1967) *Passing On*. Prentice-Hall, Englewood Cliffs, California.

Vetter, N., Jones, D. & Victor, C. (1984) Effect of health visitors working with elderly patients in general practice: a randomised controlled trial. *British Medical Journal*, **288**, 369–72.

Victor, C. & Vetter, N. (1985). The use of the health visiting service by the elderly after discharge from hospital. *Health Visitor*, **58**(4), 95–6.

Warner, U. (1984) Asking the right questions. *Nursing Times Community Outlook*, **80**(24), 214–16.

While, A. (1985) Health visiting and health experience of infants in three areas. Unpublished PhD thesis. Chelsea College, London.

# Chapter 11
# Gay men's perceptions and responses to AIDS

GRACE GETTY, *RN, BN, MN*
Associate Professor, Faculty of Nursing, Coordinator of UNB Peer Education Sexual Health Program, University of New Brunswick, Fredericton, Canada

and PHYLLIS STERN, *DNSc, RN, FAAN, NAP*
Professor and Chair, Parent-Child Nursing, School of Nursing, Indiana University, Purdue University at Indianapoplis, USA

Gay men continue to be the largest group in Canada developing AIDS. They have responded to this threat on a personal and community level. The purpose of this study was to explore the perceptions of gay men about AIDS, and how they responded to these perceptions. Data were gathered through unstructured interviews with 34 healthy gay men, from participant observations chosen from logs that described nursing interactions with gay men who had AIDS, and fieldnotes collected during AIDS education programmes with health care workers and gay men. Using constant comparative analysis, a substantive conceptual framework was developed. Trusting was identified as the basic social psychological process that determined how gay men responded to AIDS. AIDS was perceived by all gay men in this study to threaten their own health and their acceptance by society. Variables identified behaviour, ranging from denial of personal risk to taking leadership roles in organizations to fight AIDS related to the trusting theory. This theoretical explanation of gay men's responses provides direction for programmes to educate gay men about HIV-related diseases, as well as to support those who acquire the HIV virus.

## Introduction

Gay (homosexual) men continue to be the largest group developing AIDS in the western world (Update: Acquired Immunodeficiency Syndrome, 1989). At the beginning of the AIDS epidemic, the health care system perceived gay men to be the problem – a dependent patient group, whose sexual actions resulted in HIV infection (Jaffe *et al.*, 1985a, b, Marmor *et al.*, 1984, Norman 1986, Schechter *et al.*, 1985, Valdiserri *et al.*, 1984). Efforts were focused on learning about the disease, its cause and how to treat it. At the same time, the gay community recognized the threat of this disease, and gathered together to protect themselves. They did this by supporting people with AIDS and by educating gay men and others about AIDS, and how to protect themselves through safer sex (Puckett *et al.*, 1985).

The dichotomy between the health care professionals' view of gay men and their actions, and gay men's perspective of the health care professionals' inactions created a barrier that prevented them from working together to deal with necessary issues of prevention of HIV infections, and care of those affected by HIV. The purpose of this study was to learn what gay men perceive to be factors that influence their maintenance of health and how they respond to the phenomenon of AIDS. In this chapter we explain gay men's behaviours within the context of a theoretical construct that we call *trusting*. Additional variables identified will help nurses support gay men in their quest for health.

## Method

In a field-study conducted in 1985–89, grounded theory method was used to generate a theoretical framework from the data (Glaser, 1978; Hutchinson, 1986; Stern, 1980, 1985). Data were collected from three sources: (a) 34 interviews with healthy gay men; (b) participant observations selected from logs that were accounts of nursing interactions with men who had AIDS; and (c) fieldnotes gathered following AIDS education programmes with health care workers as well as gay men and lesbians. Through constant comparative analysis of data gathered in the interviews, factors were identified and hypotheses formulated. Trusting was identified as the basic social psychological process that enabled a gay man to achieve his potential, or health, and that determined how he would respond to the threat of AIDS.

### Credibility

Data from initial interviews were submitted to a Grounded Theory Seminar Group, and a sociologist for independent analysis and review of the coding process. These experts corroborated factors that were identified by the researcher, validating the accuracy of analysis. Data were chosen from nursing logs and fieldnotes after the factors had been identified from the interviews, because this theoretical sample helped to explain these factors from other perspectives.

A strength of this study was that interview data were gathered during the first year in which gay men in the study locality were diagnosed with AIDS.

As a result, the men reported current responses to AIDS, rather than retrospective data.

An attempt to obtain a representative sample of gay men was made through advertisement in a gay newsletter, special interest groups and different geographic locations. Nevertheless, all but three participants were white, Anglo-Saxon and middle class.

A possible source of bias was introduced by the fact that all the interviews were conducted by a married woman. Ross (1980) noted that gay men are fully aware of the values and beliefs of the heterosexual sphere. In a desire to 'maintain face', they might unconsciously alter reports, like those of sexual behaviour, so as to conform to their expectations of the researcher's attitudes. In this way, they might under-report their number and variety of sexual acts, especially since they wish to distance themselves from the risk of AIDS (Martin & Vance, 1984).

Nevertheless, some men described numerous varied sexual activities, choosing to 'teach' the researcher about the meaning and value of 'free' sexuality to gay men. Coates *et al.* (1986) found that there was a high degree of correlation in the responses of gay men in two different interviews when the interviewer was female. Indeed, several of the participants in this study described being able to share their thoughts and concerns more freely with female friends than with males.

The most significant evidence of credibility of this grounded theory is that data from later interviews corroborated the categories and their relationships that were identified in earlier data. After this study was completed, it was reviewed by six gay men and two lesbians, who verified the accuracy of the findings from their points of view.

Subsequent interactions with gay men have validated the factors identified. While the responses of particular study participants may have evolved, their response to AIDS has been consistent with increasing trust in themselves and others. For example, some individuals who at the time of the study refused to wear condoms now say they only practise safer sex. These men have also developed from being disclosed to only a few gay men to a virtually open lifestyle.

In this chapter we will focus on identified variables that explain a gay man's response to the threat of AIDS, within the framework of learning to trust. In the next section we present a brief description of that framework and how it was developed.

## *Trusting*

According to our data, in order to attain health a gay man must achieve the developmental tasks of unlearning myths about homosexuality, searching for gay friends and lovers, reconciling his heterosexual network with his gay identity and managing his own health. Data indicate that the critical variable of trusting in himself and others influences his ability to progress through each developmental task to the next one. As each task is achieved, his trust increases.

## Unlearning myths

Gay men reported that the task of *unlearning myths* about homosexuality is the first and most basic developmental task that follows initial ownership of a gay identity (Gonsiorek, 1988; Kus, 1985; 1986; Monteflores & Schultz, 1978; Plummer, 1989; Sprague, 1984). Almost from birth a gay man confronts myths that make up the popular stereotype of homosexuals. Gay men explained that each gay man must unlearn these mythical ideas if he is to be free to learn about and develop trust in his own identity. As he learns that such states as effeminacy, child seduction and being a sexual athlete are not necessary components of the gay life, he begins to see himself as a more trustworthy human being.

He is then free to concentrate more completely on the next developmental task, *searching for lovers and gay friends and groups* whom he can trust (Goode, 1978; Lee, 1977; Sawchuk, 1974). Gay men reported that they may differ in their attitudes towards sexual activities: while most search for a committed love relationship, they may, or may not, want a monogamous one. A proportion of gay men expressed a desire for variety as well as commitment. Data indicate that as gay men are able to accept their gayness more positively, they seek to develop a personal network of gay friends: some choose to participate in gay and lesbian associations.

After developing a personal support network of peers upon whom they can rely, gay men told us that they can begin to *reconcile their heterosexual personal network with their gay identity*. Initially, most men hide their gayness from their heterosexual friends, colleagues and family, because of their mistrust in the reactions of these heterosexuals (Goffman, 1963; Harry & DeVall, 1978; Hetrick & Martin, 1987; Sagarin & Kelly, 1980; Schur, 1979). They continue to assess this network to determine what effect disclosure of their gay identity would have. One of the challenges of this task is to maintain a realistic appraisal, rather than anticipating barriers where there are none. The tools of 'passing for straight' and disclosing their true identity are used by gay men to cope with this task of reconciliation.

## Managing health risks

The final development task we discovered is to *manage the health risks* that result from being gay. Gay men disclosed that the strong desire to remain sexually attractive results in their concern for optimal nutrition and fitness (Harry & DeVall, 1978). However, the hazards created by the stress of gayness may lead to alcoholism and drug dependence (Cabaj, 1989; Fenwick, 1982; Israelstam & Lambert, 1983; Zehner & Lewis, 1984). Sexually-transmitted diseases, especially HIV diseases, and the consequences that result from interacting with a sometimes unsympathetic health care system, were a concern for all the gay men interviewed.

Many researchers believe that the person a gay man becomes is a reaction to stigmatization by society (Jones *et al.*, 1984; Sagarin & Kelly, 1980; Reiter, 1989; Schur, 1979; Staats, 1978). According to our data, however, gay men who are able to trust themselves can make choices that allow them to achieve their potential not only in their professional and leisure activities, but also as gay men (see Fig. 11.1).

## The threat of AIDS: losing or gaining trust

All of the gay men in the study viewed the advent of AIDS as threatening: (a) their own health; (b) their gay friends and lovers; and (c) their acceptance by the heterosexual society. Perceptions of personal vulnerability to AIDS depended upon each gay man's sexual history and current practices, age, geographic location, travel patterns, network with gay men in other locations and links with persons who had developed AIDS. In large measure, even those men who had successfully transcended the developmental tasks leading to trust in themselves as gay men felt that trust weakened in the face of the calamity that is AIDS. That loss of trust was supported or refuted by their perception of personal susceptibility and society's response to themselves as potentiating the spread of AIDS.

### Links to perception of susceptibility

As the incubation period of AIDS can be as long as seven to 10 years (Goedert *et al.*, 1986), 32 of the 34 men in this study considered themselves to be vulnerable to developing AIDS. They described monitoring themselves for symptoms of AIDS, such as enlarged lymph nodes or Kaposi's sarcoma lesions (Morin & Batchelor, 1984). As Jay said, 'I look myself over ever morning like that old Chinese lady in *Hawaii* who thought she might have leprosy'.

While all these men (except for the two who had been in a monogamous relationship for 11 years) felt they could have been infected with HIV, their perception of that probability depended upon their links to susceptibility: their geographic location and mobility. For example, those men who lived in or near a large city (where several gay men had developed AIDS prior to the

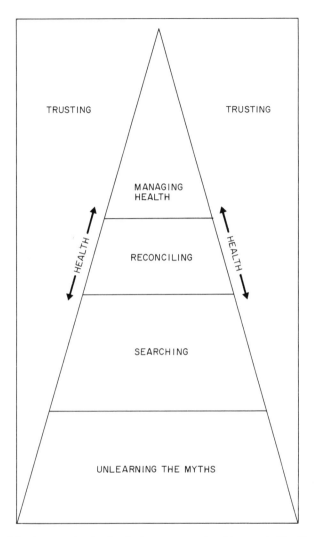

**Fig. 11.1**   Hierarchy of developmental tasks that lead to a gay man's achievement of health.

time of this study) perceived themselves to be more likely to have been infected. Their anxiety was evident in their symptoms of malaise, lethargy, reduced appetite and difficulty in sleeping, which are also early symptoms of AIDS (Bennett, 1986). This spiral of increasing anxiety followed by exacerbation of symptoms has been documented by several other researchers and clinicians (Miller & Green, 1985; Morin & Batchelor, 1984; Nichols & Ostrow, 1984). This perception of personal susceptibility was also evident in their dramatic decrease in sexual risk behaviours (Coates, 1990; Donovan & Bodsworth, 1991).

The men in this study from rural areas conceded the possibility of being infected, but in a more abstract, theoretical way. They expressed a more present danger of infection if they had visited cities with large gay communities, or if they had friends who had developed AIDS.

Rural domicile has been related to continued sexual risk behaviour (House & Walker, 1993; Kelly *et al.*, 1990). In fact, Myers *et al.* (1993) found that twice as many gay men in Atlantic Canada, a rural area of Canada, never use a condom for anal intercourse as in the national average.

**Confronting the threat of AIDS**

While all the men expressed some anxiety about their personal vulnerability to HIV, their perception of their ability to confront the threat of AIDS depended in part on prior success in achieving their developmental tasks. This confirms Clarke's (1984) contention that 'a pre-existing set of demands with which the individual is coping, renders him more likely to perceive an inability to cope with new demands or physiological stressors, and thus predisposes him to illness'.

Young men, who attended education sessions for groups of gay men and lesbians and who were still engrossed in the first developmental task of unlearning the myths about homosexuality, were likely to deny that AIDS could happen to them. John's remark was typical: 'I only go with students, so I don't have to worry'. During denial, they did not protect themselves through using safer sex techniques, such as condoms (Miller & Green, 1985). The strength of this denial was observed early in the AIDS epidemic, when pamphlets on AIDS were handed to people leaving a gay bar, who immediately tossed them to the ground.

The myth that young gay men are less likely to be infected than older gay men continues to be used as a rationale for unsafe sex (Hayes *et al.*, 1990). In fact, young gay men are more likely to have more frequent unprotected intercourse as well as to have an increased number of sexual partners (Coates, 1990; Gruer & Ssembatya-Lule, 1993; House & Walker, 1993; Myers *et al.*, 1993). They are more likely to use public cruising areas (Hayes *et al.*, 1991), and alcohol and drugs during and preceding sexual activities (Cabaj, 1989; Davidson *et al.*, 1992; Ostrow *et al.*, 1991).

*Homophobia*

Homophobic heterosexuals have suggested that the AIDS epidemic will prevent young men from acting on their gay sexual orientation because it has forged a real link between homosexual activity and death. This relationship, however, is not new for gay men. Throughout the ages, the act of making love to another man has been punishable by law, resulting in imprisonment, torture and even death (Bell, 1976; Enlow, 1984; Harry & DeVall, 1978;

Leishman, 1985; Licato, 1981). Homosexual activity also carries the threat of social death, as gay men fear being ostracized from family and friends should they be found out (Borhek, 1988; Devine, 1984; Fenwick, 1982). In spite of the fear of repercussions should their gay identity be disclosed, gay men have continued to explore and express their gayness. The fact of AIDS, and the fear of being infected with HIV, have not prevented this process. They have merely added one more cost to being gay. As Fred put it, 'It was more easy being gay; now with AIDS we may be moving back into the dark ages'.

## Locating information

In the process of unlearning the myths about homosexuality, gay men learn realities about gay culture through reading gay literature (Bell, 1976). Gay men who had unlearned the myths about homosexuality coped with the threat of AIDS by locating information, reading those articles available in the popular press and in gay magazines. As Ned said, 'I read everything I can get my hands on. We're not just a bunch of dumb nellies you know'.

At the time of the study interviews, these gay men had more knowledge about AIDS than did most health care professionals. Not only had they read prolifically, but they had accurate recall of the information. For example, the information that HIV had been found in saliva (Bennett, 1986; Curran, 1985; Gallo & Wong-Staal, 1985; Levy *et al.*, 1985) resulted in these men no longer kissing one another in greeting. They were also meticulous about not sharing glasses. Realizing that there was no evidence of HIV being transmitted via saliva (Curran, 1985), they continued to welcome friends into their homes whom they believed to be at increased risk of HIV infection. Those who had located information shared it with others, making use of a new videotape or pamphlet. In contrast, many health care workers not only remembered information about AIDS inaccurately but ostracized persons with AIDS (Douglas *et al.*, 1985; Fox, 1988; Freedman, 1988; Jenkins, 1987; Loewy, 1986; O'Donnell *et al.*, 1987; Schaffner 1985).

The gay men in this study were concerned that the information disseminated was accurate, and believed they could locate correct information in the health care system. They expressed a mistrust in the mass media, frequently using the term 'sensationalized'.

## Dignifying sexual patterns

All the men in this study asserted that they and their gay associates confronted the threat of AIDS by modifying sexual patterns, thus decreasing their amount of casual sexual activity. This is an example of Cohen & Lazarus's (1983) concept of inhibition of action as a means of coping. This assertion is corroborated by other studies of gay men (Gruer & Ssembatya-

Lule, 1993; Offir *et al.*, 1993; Puckett *et al.*, 1985; Reisenberg, 1986; Simkins & Eberhage, 1984). Mike, a chief informant, evaluated this trend, saying, 'AIDS is forcing people to either stay home or go out alone – to behave with more dignity'. Not only did Mike see decreased promiscuity as resulting in more dignity for gay men, but as facilitating the development of committed relationships. In other words, the phenomenon of AIDS has caused gay men to behave in such a way as to enhance their development of the emotional aspect of trust in one another (Driscoll, 1978; Scott, 1980). On the other hand, Kevin took the opposite view now:

> 'Overall, there has been a *drastic* change from promiscuity because of the AIDS scare. It has affected even couples because they don't have sex with each other that often any more, simply because they are blocked by the psychological worry about where their partner has been.'
>
> Getty (1987)

Kevin's belief that the threat of AIDS has magnified the mistrust between gay men, even those in committed relationships, was encapsulated by his phrase 'almost a paranoia'. The anger with which he expressed his feeling of unfairness at the loss of sexual freedom imposed by AIDS was echoed by several other men, particularly those who had been more promiscuous.

Dignifying sexual patterns is confirmed by a significant decrease in rates of gonorrhoea among gay men (Judson, 1983; Leishman, 1985; Romanowski & Brown, 1986). Unfortunately, in spite of this modifying of sexual patterns, the increasing prevalence of HIV increases the risk of each sexual encounter. This is particularly true for men who travel to areas of higher incidence of HIV infections, such as New York or Toronto (Curran, 1985; Schechter *et al.*, 1985; Stone *et al.*, 1986). Seeing the risk, George said, 'Every new affair – or even every time you have sex, it's like, is this the time it's gonna get me?'

## *Playing it safer*

Knowledge of how HIV is transmitted led about a third of this group of men to adopt safer sex practices such as using a condom for anal intercourse. These men believed that they were vulnerable to the AIDS virus, and that safer sex practices would help to protect them from HIV, if they had not already been infected, and would prevent them from transmitting it, if they had been infected. These men tended to be better educated and to be more selective about their sexual partners prior to the AIDS epidemic, than those who failed to change their sexual practices when AIDS appeared on the scene. Moreover, they were likely to be men in their late 20s and 30s, having achieved personal success in their careers, who had at least one friend with AIDS. They were also men who were more comfortable with their gay identity, having achieved the developmental tasks of unlearning the myths and searching for gay friends and lovers. Playing it safer then, depended on the developmental status of the individual in learning to trust.

Those young men who were in the process of searching for lovers and friends, were more concerned with acceptance and being popular, than the possibility they might become infected with HIV. Several expressed the fear that George did: 'If I asked someone to use a condom, he'd think there was something wrong with me' (Getty, 1987). Their fear of embarrassment, or 'loss of face' in Goffman's (1955) terminology, was so great they continued to engage in unprotected casual sex, fearing not only the reaction of this sexual partner, but also what he might say about them to other gay men. This reticence to initiate and negotiate a safer sex agreement has been found by other researchers (De Mayo & Miller, 1990; Hayes *et al.*, 1990; Morin *et al.*, 1984; Pollack *et al.*, 1990).

**Using condoms**

Even though condoms have been shown to be effective in preventing the transmission of HIV (Conant *et al.*, 1986, Stone *et al.*, 1986), their use was difficult for these gay men to adopt (Williams, 1984). They had previously viewed condoms as a heterosexual contraceptive device. Indeed, the packaging of condoms with pictures of heterosexual couples reinforced this concept, and was distasteful to these men.

One approach that has helped gay men begin to use condoms, was to present them as an erotic toy, that could enhance rather than detract from sexual pleasures (Catania *et al.*, 1989; Cochrane *et al.*, 1992; D'Eramo *et al.*, 1988). This approach was described by Bob: 'It's one of those things that can be taught on the fantasy level'. Bob's contention that the use of condoms needs to be presented as the 'in' behaviour was echoed by several men, who advocated having condom dispensers in the washroom at gay bars. For example, Bill remarked that the message condom dispensers in washrooms, would give was, 'We would like you to please take care of yourself, we don't want to lose you'.

*Maintaining health: avoiding risks*

Some men confronted the threat of AIDS by focusing on their fourth developmental task of maintaining health by avoiding risks. Bob described it well:

'I get a lot of rest; since AIDS, I've become very aware of that. I eat very well now. If I didn't work out I'd be a blimp. I practise meditation and things like that. I've tried to put myself in a very non-stressful situation.'

Getty (1987)

Bob's careful monitoring of factors that maintain his health demonstrated his feeling of self-esteem, and of being able to make changes to control his life's experiences. This was evident in several of the men in their late 20s and 30s who saw themselves as worthwhile persons. The fact that AIDS occurs more commonly among those men over 30 years of age (Peterman *et al.*, 1985; Soskoline *et al.*, 1986) means that more of their peers have succumbed to AIDS. Hence their sense of personal vulnerability is increased. Bob's consideration of factors that influence immunity, namely nutrition, rest, exercise and coping with stress, is well supported in the literature as being effective (Cecchi, 1986; Coates *et al.*, 1984; Corman, 1985; Farthing & Keusch, 1986; Martin & Vance, 1984; Morin & Batchelor, 1984; Morin *et al.*, 1984; Peterman *et al.*, 1985; Romano, 1984; Saravia, 1986; Schindler, 1985; Watson, 1984).

### Confronting screening

By law, all who test seropositive to HIV in the provinces of Nova Scotia and New Brunswick, Canada, must be reported and the records kept by government. Of the 34 men in this study, only one planned to be screened. He was an independent businessman, who lived an openly gay life citing 200 to 300 sexual partners in the past two years. He expressed terror at the thought of being infected by HIV and was so distressed that he chose to be tested for HIV immediately.

The remaining 33, however, confronted screening by being unwilling to be tested. More than half expressed a desire to know their antibody status, but they were unwilling to risk testing until their anonymity could be guaranteed. They were absolutely adamant about refusing to have their names listed in a government department. Two or three commented that the first group to be 'rounded up' and sent to concentration camps by Hitler were gay men (Haeberle, 1981; Lautmann, 1981). In fact, nearly 250 000 homosexual men were killed in Nazi concentration camps (Goode, 1978). To the men in this study, a list of gay men who are seropositive represented a powerful weapon that could be used against them. This confirms studies on the Health Belief Model that found that a person's perception of barriers to action was significant in preventing a particular health action (Chen & Tatsuoka, 1984; Kelly, 1979; Simon & Das, 1984). Myers *et al.* (1993) found that 46.1% of the gay men sampled in Atlantic Canada have still not been tested for antibodies to HIV. Anonymous testing has been found to increase the number of individuals at risk from HIV infection who seek to be tested (Hirano *et al.*, 1990; Raffi *et al.*, 1990). However, this research data has not effected any change in the way screening results have been recorded. Confronting screening illuminates gay men's loss of trust in society.

The second group who were unwilling to be screened were men who did not want to know their antibody status. Stephen said, 'It'll be hard on a person knowing [they are HIV positive], but not knowing if AIDs is going to develop'. Even Dennis, whose lover had died of AIDS a few months before our interview, said, 'They really wanted to test me – but I've said absolutely no! If I get sick – then I will go for testing, but not before!' These men feared being left alone to cope with the stress of being seropositive. They believed that systems for support of seropositive individuals, including emotional, social and intellectual support, were not currently available, but were necessary before they would confront screening by being tested for HIV. The wisdom of this belief is evident in the finding that 28.9% of those who are HIV positive in the Atlantic area have experienced rejection by other gay men following their disclosure, compared to 10.7% in the rest of Canada (Myers *et al.*, 1993).

## Confronting the blame

All of the men in this study were confronting the blame for the AIDS epidemic. All believed that AIDS would lead to an escalation of homophobia (a fear and hatred of gay individuals) resulting in more repressive social conditions for gay men and lesbians. Fifteen per cent of these men even believed that AIDS was being allowed to decimate the gay male population as a plot hatched by 'straight society'. All who believed this were under 30 years of age and had expressed extreme mistrust of heterosexuals, based on experiences of having been publicly humiliated and harassed. For example, Jack said, 'It's almost a genocidal ploy because they are very lax with getting treatment and with research. They don't seem to care for AIDS patients very much.' Jack's comments demonstrate his degree of anger and mistrust of the established political system. However, his statements are no more vehement than those of groups such as Physicians Against AIDS and conservative fundamentalists, such as the cleric Gerry Falwell, who have lobbied politicians to return homosexuality to the criminal code (Batchelor, 1984; Korcok, 1985; Panem, 1984; Patten, 1985).

While just 15% of the study population believed that there was a conspiracy to allow AIDS to eliminate gay men, 94% believed that the negligence of public health departments in not dispensing adequate economic and personnel resources to combat AIDS was due to a lack of valuing gay men, and the other stigmatized risk groups. Kevin commented, 'The key element is information not being passed on. Nobody is getting any information from public health. To me personally it gives further distrust of the system.' Several of these men contended that the news of Rock Hudson's development of AIDS would increase the value attributed to its victims. This they thought would lead to more effort to overcome AIDS. This belief was corroborated when millions of dollars were subsequently channelled into research, education and support services, both by governments and private individuals. More recent data from gay men indicate that these activities have helped to restore their trust in themselves and in society.

## Forming and using social support networks

The extensive social network of gay men has facilitated transmission of HIV, not only within a particular community, but also from one geographic location to another (Altman, 1986; Fettner & Check, 1984; Klovdahl, 1985; Peterman *et al.*, 1985). The tendency for gay men to migrate to large urban centres after identifying their gayness, as well as their predilection to travel extensively, has provided a means for transportation of HIV infection from one area to another. About 75% of the gay men in this study knew at least one person with AIDS. The same links are now being used as channels of communication to transmit information about AIDS. They are using social support networks to fight AIDS.

In each geographic location, one or two men became the central figures, taking responsibility for obtaining and disseminating literature on AIDS to local gay men. These men had accomplished the developmental task of assuming leadership roles. This provision of information, a cognitive function of social support, was perceived by other gay men as providing a source of power to enable them to assume responsibility for their own health and safety (Kelner, 1985; Stevens, 1983).

In particular, the participants in this study worried about those closeted gays who were even reluctant to read accounts of AIDS in the popular press. Having been closeted themselves in the past, these gay men were sensitive to the feelings and reactions of those who continue to hide. They believed that closeted gay men are concerned about AIDS, but that the threat of disclosure was more immediately relevant to them than the future possibility of illness. These closeted men had been unable to transcend developmental tasks towards trusting. Several suggestions of methods to deliver information about AIDS and safer sex practices to those closeted gay men were made, including a telephone AIDS-Line, posters in public washrooms and brochures mailed to every household.

### Change in attitude

The concern for other gay men shown by these men demonstrates the profound change in the attitude of gay men towards the well-being of their peers since the advent of AIDS. Bill clearly demonstrated this change. At first, when he described the entry of young gay men to the gay club, and their involvement with 'the wrong group' and drugs and alcohol, he was content to observe what was happening. He denied feeling any responsibility to intervene or redirect these youths. However, after one of his friends died with AIDS he became concerned about the well-being of other gay men, advocating safer sex practices through passing out pamphlets and showing videos about AIDS.

This concern for other gay men led Bill and other gay men to organize a committee to use social support networks by providing help for those who became infected with HIV and developed AIDS. For example, they visited persons with AIDS (PWAs) who were in hospital, and maintained emotional support for these men throughout their illness, even when they had not known them prior to their hospitalization (Kelner, 1985).

## Solidarity

The experience of using social support networks to help individuals who were receiving health care for HIV infection has led to a growing solidarity in the gay community (Lopez & Getzel, 1984). Both gay men – and the rest of society – have seen evidence of the worth of each individual as they volunteered to help ameliorate the effects of AIDS for others (Cecchi, 1984). In return, the sense of control and having power over some aspect of what may occur, helped to maintain the health of those groups of gay men who were volunteering their time (Kelner, 1985).

With the support of one another, some gay men have stepped into the open, speaking to groups of people about being gay and their response to AIDS. While this disclosure took great courage, it was met by acceptance and support from many heterosexuals. As a result, gay men's *trust* in themselves, as well as of health care professionals, has been enhanced. In fact, the leadership shown by gay men has demonstrated achievement of their potential toward trusting: a higher level of health than they would have expected prior to the AIDS epidemic (see Fig. 11.2).

## *Nursing implications of learning to trust*

Transmission of information about HIV infection has been the primary intervention used in most AIDS education programmes (Solomon & Dejong, 1986). This study helps to explain some of the reasons why all gay men do not adopt or maintain safer sex behaviours. Until health education programmes help gay men to achieve their developmental tasks of unlearning the myths about homosexuality, by including information about the positive

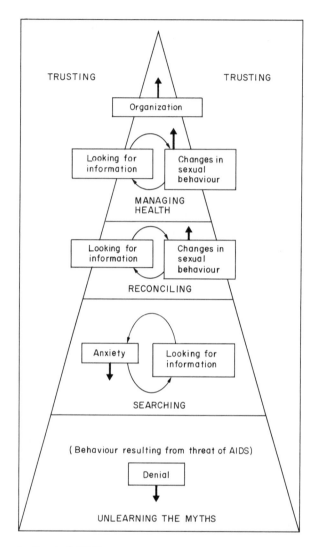

**Fig. 11.2**   Response to the threat of AIDS.

acceptance of homosexuality, they will not reach gay men who are beginning to explore their sexual identity. Instead, they will continue to preach to the converted, those who have learned to trust themselves and their gay peers and who have already changed to safer sex. Research on other factors that influence the adoption and maintenance of safer sex behaviours is imperative. The information that many gay men continue to have difficulty negotiating a safer sex agreement will provide an important area to consider in a nursing care plan. Both through problem solving in a helping relationship, and the use of such techniques as role-playing, nurses can help these men find their own method to negotiate safer sex. Progress in this changing behaviour will be enhanced when continuity of care is maintained. This factor implies that clinics should be organized so that particular clients are assigned to the case-load of a particular nurse.

Nurses need to recognize and applaud the leadership shown by gay men and lesbians in the war against AIDS. A collaborative relationship with these individuals is important if prevention is to be effective. The information about particular natural leaders, or central figures, who are able to influence their peers is useful to nurses who wish to establish health education and promotion programmes. These men have access to this closeted group of gay men and lesbians, and can make such programmes possible (D'Aquila & Vallance, 1982; Galaskiewicz & Shatin, 1981).

The demands of gay men to be equal partners in the fight against AIDS must be recognized and encouraged. The knowledge that gay men expect to be discriminated against by heterosexuals, as well as to be blamed for AIDS, helps nurses understand their anger and defensiveness when dependent on others for care. The personal networks among gay men in which they share their mutual fear of AIDS, provide avenues through which education and other services can be delivered (Kelner, 1985).

## Educational programmes

In view of the fact that gay men locate information about HIV infection and how they can maintain their immune status, it is important that nurses tailor their educational programmes to their client's specific need for information. For example, while alcoholism and drug dependency are common problems among gay men, increased intake of alcohol, as well as stress and malnutrition decrease the T4 cells and harm their immune systems (Watson, 1984) at the very time HIV threatens their T4 cells. It is, accordingly, important for the nurse to teach these clients about these physiological reactions and how to limit them, such as relaxation exercises, Live and Let Live groups or Alcoholic Anonymous groups for gay clientele.

## Shared efforts and mutual goals

In this study we found that although AIDS has increased the mistrust in the safety of sexual activities between gay men, it has drawn them together in other ways. As they have organized themselves to deal with the threat of AIDS, they are finding new satisfactions in shared efforts to achieve mutual goals. AIDS has, in fact, given them more common interests on which to build their relationships. The long-term support that is necessary for those individuals who learn they are seropositive for HIV can be provided through the development of support groups. Before these are adopted, we need to study the ways in which support groups have developed in other places, and their impact on gay men's personal networks. For example, we need to know more about: (a) the density and qualities of the individual's personal network and support system; (b) the characteristics of men who became involved in support groups; (c) the effect on the group members of the development of AIDS in one member; and (d) how support groups relate to the formal organization of gay individuals and use power to deal with issues, such as discrimination against AIDS patients and public debate.

## Conclusion

This study gives nurses information that will help them care for gay men who are infected with HIV and develop AIDS. However, it also demonstrates the need for nurses to support gay men who are healthy to accomplish their developmental tasks so as to attain holistic health, or high level wellness. Nurses with knowledge of the variables of how gay men facing the threat of AIDS gain or lose trust about their links to susceptibility, about confronting the threat of AIDS, locating information, dignifying sexual patterns, playing it safer, maintaining health, avoiding risks, confronting screening, confronting blame and their way of using social support networks to fight AIDS, can make use of these variables to support gay men in their positive health behaviours and provide relevant interventions where these behaviours are absent. As Flaherty (1985) said, 'The phenomena with which nurses are concerned are people's health seeking and coping behaviours as they strive to attain health'.

## References

Altman, D. (1986) *AIDS and the New Puritanism*. Pluto, London.

Batchelor, W. (1984) AIDS: a public health and psychological emergency. *American Psychologist*, **39**(11), 1279–84.

Bell, R. (1976) *Social Deviance: A Substantive Analysis*. Irwin-Dorsey, Georgetown.

Bennett, J. (1986) AIDS: what we should know. *American Journal of Nursing*, **86**, 1016–28.

Borhek, M.H. (1988) Helping gay and lesbian adolescents and their families. *Journal of Adolescent Health Care*, **9**, 123–8.

Cabaj, R. (1989) AIDS and chemical dependency: special issues and treatment barriers for gay and bisexual men. *Journal of Psychoactive Drugs*, **21**(4), 387–93.

Catania, J., Coates, T. Kegeles, S., Ekstrand, M., Guydish, J., & Bye, L. (1989) Implications of the AIDS risk-reduction model for the gay community: the importance of sexual enjoyment and help-seeking behaviors. In *Primary Prevention of AIDS* (eds V. Mays, G. Albee & S. Schneider), pp. 242–61. Sage, London.

Cecchi, R.L. (1984) Stress prodrome to immune deficiency. *Annals of New York Academy of Science*, **371**, 286–9.

Cecchi, R.L. (1986) When the system fails. *American Journal of Nursing*, 45–7.

Chen, M. & Tatsuoka, M. (1984) The relationship between American women's preventive dental behavior and dental health beliefs. *Social Science and Medicine*, **19**, 971–8.

Clarke, M. (1984) Stress and coping: constructs for nursing. *Journal of Advanced Nursing*, **9**, 3–13.

Coates, T. (1990) Strategies for modifying sexual behavior for primary and secondary prevention of HIV disease. *Journal of Consulting and Clinical Psychology*, **58**(1), 57–69.

Coates, T.J., Temoshok, L. & Mandel, J. (1984). Psychosocial research is essential to understanding and treating AIDS. *American Psychologist*, 1309–14.

Cochrane, S., Mays, V., Ciarletta, J., Caruso, C. & Mallon (1992) Efficacy of the theory of reasoned behavior in predicting AIDS-related sexual risk reduction among gay men. *Journal of Applied Social Psychology*, **22**(19), 1481–1501.

Cohen, F. & Lazarus, R.S. (1983) Coping and adaptation in health and illness. In *Handbook of Health, Health Care and the Health Professions* (ed D. Mechanic). Free Press, New York.

Conant, M., Hardy, D. Sernatinger, J., Spicer, D. & Levy, J. (1986) Condoms prevent transmission of AIDS-associated retrovirus. *Journal of American Medical Association*, **255**(13), 1706.

Corman, L.C. (1985) Effects of specific nutrients on the immune response, selected clinical applications. *Medical Clinics of North America*, **69**(4), 759–86.

Curran, J. (1985) The epidemiology and prevention of the Acquired Immunodeficiency Syndrome. *Annals of Internal Medicine*, **103**, 657–62.

D'Aquila, A.R. & Vallance, T.R. (1982) The helping community: issues in the evaluation of a preventive intervention to promote informal helping. *Journal of Community Psychology*, **10**, 199–208.

Davidson, S., Dew, M., Penkower, L., Becker, J., Kingsley, L. & Sullivan, P. (1992) Substance use and sexual behavior among homosexual men at risk for HIV infection: psychosocial moderators. *Psychology and Health*, **7**, 259–72.

D'Eramo, J. Quadlands, M., Shatts, W., Schuman, R. & Jacobs, R. (1988) *The '800 men' project: a systematic evaluation of AIDS prevention programs demonstrating the efficacy of erotic, sexually explicit safer sex education on gay and bisexual men at risk for AIDS.* Paper presented at the Fourth International Conference on AIDS, Stockholm, Sweden.

De Mayo, M. & Miller, R. (1990) *Reinforcing safer sex and preventing relapse to high risk behaviors among gay men.* Paper presented at the Sixth International Conference on AIDS, San Francisco.

Devine, J. (1984) A systematic inspection of affectional preference orientation and the family of origin. *Social Work*, **29**, 9–17.

Donovan, B. & Bodsworth, N. (1991) *Homosexually acquired gonorrhea is limited as a marker for relapse into HIV risk behavior.* Paper presented at the Seventh International Conference on AIDS, Florence.

Douglas, C.J., Kalman, C.M. & Kalman, T.P. (1985) Homophobia among physicians and nurses: an empirical study. *Hospital and Community Psychiatry*, **36**(2), 1309–11.

Driscoll, J.W. (1978) Trust and participation in organizational decision making as predictors of satisfaction. *Academy of Management Journal*, **21**(1), 44–56.

Enlow, R. (1984) Special session. *Annals of New York Academy of Sciences*, **371**, 290–311.

Farthing, M.J. & Keusch, G.T. (1986) Gut parasites: nutritional and immunological interaction. In *Nutrition, Disease Resistance and Immune Function* (ed. R.R. Watson), pp. 87–112. Marcell Dekker, New York.

Fenwick, R.D. (1982) *The Advocate Guide to Gay Health*, Alyson, Boston.

Fettner, A.G. & Check, W.A. (1984) *The Truth About AIDS: Evolution of an Epidemic.* Holt, Rinehart & Winston, New York.

Flaherty (1985) Ethical issues. In *Community Health Nursing in Canada* (eds M. Stewart, J. Ennes, S. Searl & C. Smillie). Gage, Toronto.

Fox, D.M. (1988) The politics of physicians' responsibility in epidemics: a note on history. *Hastings Center Report*, **18**, 5–10.

Freedman, B. (1988) Health professions, codes, and the right to refuse to treat HIV-infectious patients. *Hastings Center Report*, **18**, 20–25.

Galaskiewicz, J. & Shatin, D. (1981) Leadership and networking among neighbourhood human service organizations. *Administrative Science Quarterly*, **26**, 434–48.

Gallo, R.C. & Wong-Staal, F. (1985) A human T-lymphotropic retrovirus (HTLV-III) as the cause of the Acquired Immunodeficiency Syndrome. *Annals of Internal Medicine*, **103**, 679–89.

Getty, G.A. (1987) Toward trust: Prerequisite for gay health in a world with AIDS. Unpublished masters thesis. Dalhousie University, Hallifax, Nova Scotia.

Gerald, G. (1989) What can we learn from the gay community's response to the AIDS crisis? *Journal of the American Medical Association*, **81**(4), 449–52.

Glaser, B.C. (1978) *Theoretical Sensitivity*. The Sociology Press, Mill Valley, California.

Goedert, J.J., Biggar, R., Weiss, J., Eyster, M., Melbye, M., Wilson, S. *et al.* (1986) Three year incidence of AIDS in five cohorts of HTLV-III infected risk group members, *Science*, **231**, 992–5.

Goffman, E. (1955) On face-work: an analysis of ritual elements in social interaction. *Psychiatry*, **18**, 213–31.

Goffman, E. (1963) *Stigma: Notes on the Management of a Spoiled Identity*. Prentice-Hall, Englewood Cliffs, New Jersey.

Gonsiorek, J.C. (1988) Mental health issues of gay and lesbian adolescents. *Journal of Adolescent Health Care*, **9**,114–22.

Goode, E. (1978) *Deviant Behavior: An Interactionist Approach*. Prentice-Hall, Englewood Cliffs, New Jersey.

Gruer, L. & Ssembatya-Lule, G. (1993) Sexual behavior and the use of the condom by men attending gay bars and clubs in Glasgow and Edinburgh. *International Journal of STD and AIDS*, **4**, 95–8.

Haeberle, E. (1981) Stigmata of degeneration: prison markings in Nazi concentration camps. In *Historical Perspectives on Homosexuality* (eds S. Licato & R. Peterson), pp. 56–73. Haworth Press, New York.

Harry, J. & DeVall, W. (1978) *The Social Organization of Gay Males*. Praeger, New York.

Hayes, R., Kegeles, S. & Coates, T. (1990) *Why are young gay men engaging in high rates of unsafe sex?* Paper presented at the Sixth International Conference on AIDS, San Francisco.

Hayes, R. Kegeles, S. & Coates, T. (1991) *Understanding the high rates of HIV-risk taking among young gay and bisexual men: the young men's survey*. Paper presented at the Seventh International Conference on AIDS, Florence.

Hetrick, E.S. & Martin, A.D. (1987) Developmental issues and their resolution for gay and lesbian adolescents. *Journal of Homosexuality*, **13**, 25–43.

Hirano, D., Englender, S., Fleming, K., England, B., Spry, J., Komatsu, K., Moore, M., & Sands, L. (1990) *Impact of a 1989 testing change in Arizona: preliminary analysis*. Paper presented at the Sixth International Conference on AIDS, San Francisco.

House, R., & Walker, C. (1993) Preventing AIDS through education. *Journal of Counselling and Development*, **71**, 282–9.

Hutchinson, S. (1986) Grounded theory: the method. In *Nursing Research: A Qualitative Perspective*. (eds P.L. Munhall & C.J. Oiler), pp. 111–129. Appleton–Century–Croft, Norwalk, Connecticut.

Israelstam, S. & Lambert, S. (1983) Homosexuality as a cause of alcoholism: a historical review. *The International Journal of the Addictions*, **18**(8), 1085–1107.

Jaffe, H., Darrow, W., Echenberg, D., O'Mally, P., Cetchell, J., Kalyanaraman V. *et al.* (1985a). The Acquired Immunodeficiency Syndrome in a cohort of homosexual men. *Annals of Internal Medicine*, **103**, 210–14.

Jaffe, H., Hardy, A., Morgan, M. & Darrow, W. (1985b) The Acquired Immunodeficiency Syndrome in gay men. *Annals of Internal Medicine*, **103**, 662–4.

Jenkins, K. (1987) Silence could mean a difference between life and death for an injured AIDS patient. *The Medical Post*, **23**(40), 2.

Jones, E., Farina, A., Markers, H., Miller, P., Scott, R. & French, R. (1984) *Social Stigma: The Psychology of Marked Relationships*. W.H. Freedman, New York.

Judson, F. (1983) Fear of AIDS and gonorrhoea rates in homosexual men. *Lancet*, **2**, 159–60.

Kelly, P.T. (1979) Breast self-examinations: who does them and why. *Journal of Behavioral Medicine*, **2**, 31–8.

Kelly, J., St Lawrence, J., Brasfield, T., Stevenson, Y., Diaz, Y. & Hauth, A. (1990) AIDS risk behavior patterns among gay men in small southern cities. *American Journal of Public Health*, **80**, 1–2.

Kelner, M. (1985) Community support networks: current issues. *Canadian Journal of Public Health*, **76** (suppl. 1) 69–70.

Klovdahl, A.S. (1985) Social networks and the spread of infectious diseases: the AIDS example. *Social Science and Medicine*, **21**(11), 1203–16.

Korcok, M. (1985) AIDS hysteria: a contagious side effect. *Canadian Medical Association Journal*, **133**, 1241–8.

Kus, R. (1985) Stages of coming out: an ethnographic approach. *Western Journal of Nursing Research*, **7**(2), 177–98.

Kus, R.J. (1986) From grounded theory to clinical practice: cases from gay studies research. In *From Practice to Grounded Theory: Qualitative Research in Nursing* (eds. W.C. Chenitz & J.M. Swanson), pp. 227–40. Addison-Wesley, Don Mills, Ontario.

Lautmann, R. (1981) The pink triangle: the persecution of homosexual males in concentration camps in Nazi Germany. In *Historical Perspectives on Homosexuality* (eds S. Licato & R. Peterson), pp. 42–55. Haworth, New York.

Lee, J. (1977) Going public: a study in the sociology of homosexual liberation. *Journal of Homosexuality*, **3**(1), 49–78.

Leishman, K. (1985) A crisis in public health. *The Atlantic*, **253**, 18–41.

Levy, J., Kaminsky, L., Morrow, J., Steimer, K., Lucius, P., Dina, D. *et al.* (1985) Infection by the retrovirus associated with the Acquired Immunodeficiency Syndrome. *Annals of Internal Medicine*, **103**, 694–9.

Licato, S. (1981) The homosexual rights movement in the United States: a traditionally over-looked area of American history. In *Historical Perspectives on Homosexuality* (eds S. Licato & R. Peterson), pp. 1–23. Haworth, New York.

Loewy, E.H. (1986) E.H. (1986) AIDS and the physicians fear of contagion. *Chest*, **89**(3), 325–6.

Lopez, D. & Getzel, G. (1984) Helping gay AIDS patients in crisis. *Social Casework*, **65**, 387–94.

Marmor, M., El-Sadr, W., Zolla-Pazner, S., Lazaro, C., Stahl, R.E. & William, D. (1984) Immunologic abnormalities among male homosexuals in New York City: changes over time. *Annals of New York Academy of Sciences*, **371**, 312–19.

Martin, J.L. & Vance, C.S. (1984) Behavioral and psychosocial factors in AIDS, methodological and substantive issues. *American Psychologist*, **39**, 1303–8.

Miller, D. & Green, J. (1985) Psychological support and counselling for patients with acquired immune deficiency syndrome (AIDS), *Genitourinary Medicine*, **61**, 273–8.

Monteflores, C. & Schultz, S.J. (1978) Coming out: similarities and differences for lesbians and gay men. *Journal of Social Issues*, **34**(3), 59–72.

Morin, S.F. & Batchelor, W.F. (1984) Responding to the psychological crisis of AIDS. *Public Health Reports*, **99**(1), 4–9.

Morin, S.F., Charles, K.A. & Malyon, A.K. (1984) The psychological impact of AIDS on gay men. *American Psychologist*, **39**(11), 1288–93.

Myers, T., Godin, G., Calzavara, L., Lambert, J., & Locker, D. (1993) *The Canadian Survey of Gay and Bisexual Men and HIV Infection: Men's Survey*. The Canadian AIDS Society, Ottawa.

Nichols, J. & Ostrow, D. (1984) *Psychiatric Implications of Acquired Immune Deficiency Syndrome*. American Psychiatric Press, Washington.

Norman, C. (1986) AIDS priority fight goes to court. *Science*, **231**, 1063.

O'Donnell, L., O'Donnell, C.R. & Pleck, J.H. (1987) Psychosocial responses of hospital workers to acquired immune deficiency syndrome (AIDS). *Journal of Applied Social Psychology*, **17**(3), 269–85.

Offir, J., Fisher, J., Williams, S. & Fisher, W. (1993) Reasons for inconsistent AIDS-preventive behaviors among gay men. *The Journal of Sex Research*, **30**(1), 62–9.

Ostrow, D., Beltran, E. Chmiel, J., Wesch, J. & Joseph, J. (1991) *Predictors of volatile nitrate use among the Chicago MACS Cohort of homosexual men.* Paper presented at the Eighth International Conference on AIDS, Amsterdam.

Panem, S. (1984) AIDS, public policy and biomedical research. *Chest*, **85**(3), 416–22.

Patten, C. (1985) The ethics of AIDS research – weighing the risk. *The Official Newsletter of the NCGSTDS*, **6**(4), 34–5.

Peterman, T.A., Drotman, D.P. & Curran, J.W. (1985) Epidemiology of the Acquired Immunodeficiency Syndrome (AIDS), *Epidemiological Reviews*, **7**, 1–21.

Pollack, L., Ekstrand, M., Stall, R. & Coates, T. (1990) *Current reasons for having unsafe sex among gay men in San Francisco: the AIDS Behavioural Research Project.* Paper presented at the Sixth International Conference on AIDS, San Francisco.

Plummer, K. (1989) Lesbian and gay youth in England. *Journal of Homosexuality*, **17**(3–4), 195–223.

Puckett, S., Bart, M. & Amory, J. (1985) Self-reported behavioral change among gay and bisexual men – San Francisco. *Morbidity and Mortality Weekly Report*, **34**(40), 613–14.

Raffi, F., Milpied, B., Charonnat, M., Billaud, M., Ponge, A. & Litoux, P. (1990) *Free and anonymous HIV testing center of Nantes, France: 1989 experience.* Paper presented at the Sixth International Conference on AIDS, San Francisco.

Reisenberg, D. (1986) AIDS prompted behavior changes reported. *Journal of American Medical Association*, **255**(2), 171–2.

Reiter, L. (1989) Sexual orientation, sexual identity, and the question of choice. *Clinical Social Work Journal*, **17**(2), 138–50.

Romano, J.L. (1984) Stress management and wellness: reaching beyond the counselor's office. *Personnel and Guidance Journal*, **62**, 533–7.

Romanowski, B. & Brown, J. (1986) AIDS and changing sexual behavior. *Canadian Medical Association Journal*, **134**, 533–7.

Ross, M.W. (1980) Retrospective distortion in homosexual research. *Archives of Sexual Behaviour*, **9**, 523–31.

Sagarin, E. & Kelly, R (1980) Sexual deviance and labelling perspectives. In *The Labelling of Deviance* (ed W. Grove), pp. 347–75. Sage, London.

Saravia, N.G. (1986) Measles, immunity and malnutrition. In *Nutrition, Disease Resistance and Immune Function* (ed R.R. Watson), pp. 113–48. Marcel Dekker, New York.

Sawchuck, P. (1974) Becoming a homosexual. In *Decency and Deviance* (eds J. Haas & B. Shaffir). McLelland & Stewart, Toronto.

Schaffner, B. (1985) Reactions to persons with AIDS. *Academy Forum*, **29**(2), 10–13.

Schechter, M., Boyko, W. & Jeffries, E. (1985) The Vancouver AIDS Study. *Canadian Medical Association Journal*, **133**.

Schindler, B.A. (1985) Stress, affective disorders and immune function. *Medical Clinics of North America*, **69**(3), 585–95.

Schur, E. (1979) *Interpreting Deviance.* Harper & Row, New York.

Scott, C.L. (1980) Interpersonal trust: a comparison of attitudinal and situational factors. *Human Relations*, **33**(11), 805–12.

Simkins, L. & Eberhage, M.G. (1984) Attitudes towards AIDS, Herpes II & toxic shock syndrome. *Psychological Reports*, **55**, 779–86.

Simon, K. & Das, A. (1984) An application of the health belief model towards educational diagnosis for V.D. education. *Health Education Quarterly*, **11**(4), 403–18.

Solomon, M.Z. & Dejong, W. (1986) Recent sexually transmitted disease prevention efforts and their implications for AIDS health education. *Health Education Quarterly*, **13**(4), 301–16.

Soskoline, C.L., Coates, R.A. & Sears, A.G. (1986) Characteristics of a male homosexual/bisexual study population in Toronto/Canada. *Canadian Journal of Public Health*, **77**, 12–16.

Sprague, C.A. (1984) Male homosexuality in western culture: the dilemma of identity and subculture in historical research. *Journal of Homosexuality*, **10**(3/4), 29–43.

Staats, G. (1978) *Images of Deviant's Stereotypes and their Importance for Labeling Deviant Behavior.* University Press, Washington.

Stern, P.N. (1980) Grounded theory methodology: its uses and processes. *Image*, **12**(1), 20–23.

Stern, P.N. (1985) Using grounded theory method in nursing research. In *Qualitative Research Methods in Nursing* (ed. M.M. Leininger), pp. 149–60. Grunz & Stratton, Orlando.

Stevens, K.R. (1983) *Power and Influence: A Sourcebook for Nurses. John Wiley, Toronto.*

Stone, K.M., Grimes, D.A. & Magder, L.S. (1986) Primary prevention of sexually transmitted diseases. *Journal of American Medical Association,* **25**(13), 1763–66.

Update: Acquired Immunodeficiency Syndrome (1989) *Morbidity and Mortality Weekly Reports,* **38**(24), 423–33.

Valdiserri, R.D., Brandon, W.R. & Lyter, D.W. (1984) AIDS surveillance and health education: use of previously described risk factors to identify high-risk homosexuals. *Public Health Reports,* **74**(3), 259–60.

Watson, R. (1984) Stress caused by dietary changes: Corticosteroid production, a partial explanation for immunosuppression in the malnourished. In *Nutrition, Disease Resistance and Immune Function* (ed. R.R. Watson), pp. 283–84. Marcel Dekker, New York.

Williams, D. (1984) The prevention of AIDS by modifying sexual behavior. *Annals of New York Academy of Sciences,* **371**, 283–5.

Zehner, M.A. & Lewis, J. (1984) Homosexuality and alcoholism: social and developmental perspectives. *Journal of Homosexuality,* **10**, 75–89.

# Chapter 12
# Feminist research: definitions, methodology, methods and evaluation

CHRISTINE WEBB, *BA, MSc, PhD, SRN, RSCN, RNT*
Professor of Nursing, University of Manchester, Stopford Building, Oxford Road,
Manchester M13 9PT, England

The literature relating to feminist research both within and beyond nursing is reviewed in this chapter. Feminist research is located within a post-positivist paradigm, and various definitions are considered. The distinctive methodological approach of feminist research is discussed, and interviewing and ethnography are evaluated as suitable methods for use in feminist research. Oakley's (1981) paper on interviewing women is subjected to criticism. A final section examines attempts by three sets of writers to propose evaluation criteria for feminist research. The review concludes that a number of paradoxes and dilemmas in feminist research have yet to be resolved.

## Introduction

Some years have now passed since the first discussion of feminist research methodology was published in a British nursing journal (Webb, 1984). Feminist approaches to research have developed enormously since then and it is therefore timely to update this review of the literature, which includes critiques of some of the more influential early British work, particularly Oakley's now classic paper 'Interviewing women: a contradiction in terms' (Oakley, 1981).

This review will consider definitions of feminist research, before going on to examine methods used. A general consideration of methods will precede a discussion of interviewing and ethnography in particular. Issues of validity and evaluating feminist research will be the final topics.

## What is feminist research?

Feminist research is based on a particular theory of knowledge, or epistemology, and it is from this that its methodology and methods are derived

(Campbell & Bunting, 1991). Methodology refers to 'a theory and analysis of how research does or should proceed' (Harding, 1987), whereas methods are ways of gathering data. Thus feminist research is not simply the study of women, nor is it enough that it is done by women. For McCormack (1981) it involves 'a set of principles of inquiry: a feminist philosophy of science'.

The crucial distinction is that feminist research is carried out *for* women. Klein (1983) states:

'I define research for women as research that tries to take women's needs, interests and experiences into account and aims at being instrumental in improving women's lives in one way or another.'

For Wilkinson (1986) feminist research is research on women and for women, 'giving priority to female experience and developing theory which is firmly situated in this experience'. It therefore depends on the development of a different relationship between researcher and researched from that in traditional approaches. Wise (1987) takes this point even further in stating that feminist research should be 'concerned with women's oppression' and should be 'located within a model where the power imbalance (between researcher and researched) can be broken down'.

## Concerned with values

MacPherson (1983) also considers that there should be an essential focus on 'women's oppression and a concern for improving their state'. Feminist research should therefore be 'concerned with values', should focus on 'women-related research questions', should analyse 'the condition of women's lives', and should be 'grounded in actual experiences closely related to social change'. In addition, research findings should be made available to those who have taken part in the research and to women in general, for unless this is done they have no possibility of using the findings in their personal lives.

Perhaps the most comprehensive definition is incorporated within Bernhard's (1984) eight criteria for feminist research, which are that:

(1) The researcher is a woman.
(2) Feminist methodology is used, including researcher–subject interaction, non-hierarchical research relationships, expressions of feelings, and concern for values.
(3) The research has the potential to help its subjects.
(4) The focus is on the experience of women.
(5) It is a study of women.
(6) The words 'feminism' or 'feminist' are actually used.

(7) Feminist literature is cited.

(8) The research is reported using non-sexist language.

Using these criteria, Bernhard (1984) reviewed 90 nursing research reports published in two five-year periods in *Nursing Research*. She found no study meeting all eight criteria, and four or fewer criteria were fulfilled in 73 reports. She concludes that little feminist research is being carried out in nursing, or alternatively that it is not being published.

## Can men do feminist research?

Harding (1987) defines feminist research as being done for women and from the perspective of their experiences. She also requires that:

> 'the inquirer her/himself must be placed in the same critical plane as the overt subjective matter, thereby recovering the entire research process for scrutiny.'

As long as this condition is fulfilled it is possible for men to do feminist research, in her view. McCormack (1981) also points out that research on women by women is not necessarily feminist.

However, most contributors to the debate dissent strongly from this position. For example, Mies (1983) states that:

> 'Women social scientists are better equipped to make a comprehensive study of the exploited groups. Men often do not have the experiential knowledge, and therefore lack empathy, the ability for identification and because of this they also lack social and sociological imagination.'

Kremer (1990) also excludes men from being feminist researchers. She discusses the evolution of women's studies courses in educational institutions, and notes that 'new female spaces and meanings and their recognition are hard-won'. It has been difficult to establish such areas of study as legitimate and valid, and the maintenance of 'the integrity and necessity of women-only space is elemental to feminism'. If men were considered able to do feminist research there would be a danger of it becoming 'yet another discourse in which men speak to men about women', as has traditionally been the case in social science.

### Not gender studies

Evans (1990) shares this position, and argues that women's studies should continue to exist and not be replaced by gender studies as has been the case in some educational settings. She holds that it is essential to ensure a 'continued use of a term which maintains a focus on sexual difference' because 'it is not as if sexism and/or sexist understanding had disappeared from the world of learning'.

This belief is shared by Kremer (1990), who also thinks that men who have an appreciation of feminist issues would realize their incompatibility with feminist research. She states:

> 'We cannot afford to lose these (women's) spaces, these meanings, this power; besides, no truly feminist man would try and colonize these meanings, for how could such an enterprise possibly be feminist?'

The overwhelming majority of writers, therefore, take the view that men cannot take part in feminist research as researchers. However, because her definition of feminist research involves a focus on women's oppression, and because this oppression is by men, Wise (1987) takes the stance that men should be included in feminist research as subjects of study.

## *Values and feminist research*

Lather (1988) locates feminist research firmly within the post-positivism or post-modernism debate. This debate emerges from a recognition of the 'inadequacy of positivist assumptions in the face of human complexity', and the results in 'questioning of the lust for authoritative accounts'. Post-modernists recognize that it is no longer possible for a single methodology to be appropriate to study all topics, and call for a recognition of the limitations of traditional ways of 'doing science' which accepts its limitations, acknowledging that 'ways of knowing are inherently culture-bound and perspectival'.

Post-modernists, according to Lather (1988) favour change-enhancing, advocacy approaches to inquiry which 'empower the researched and contribute to the generation of change-enhancing social theory'. Feminist methodology fits with this approach because of its emphasis on critique of women's traditional position in society, its call for research relationships to be non-hierarchical, and its emphasis on being for women and being intended to facilitate change. Thus, feminist research like all post-modernist approaches should be 'praxis-oriented ... critical and empowering ... openly committed to critiquing the status quo and building a more just society' (Lather, 1988).

### Value-neutral social science

Hesse (1980) also believes that there is an increasing rejection of so-called value-neutral social science because it is 'at best unrealizable, and at worst self-deceptive, and is being replaced by social sciences based on explicit ideologies'. Feminism would be included as one of these ideologies.

These critiques of traditional scientific approaches are particularly aimed at assumptions of objectivity and the separation of researcher and researched. Du Bois (1983) accepts these critiques, and claims that:

> 'feminist scholarship reveals a different animating assumption; that the knower and known are of the same universe, that they are *not* separate.' (Emphasis in original).

Post-positivism encompasses critical theory, which had its origins in German philosophy and the work of Adorno (1976), Habermas (1976) and Bernstein (1983), among others. Feminist and critical approaches share many assumptions, but they also have distinct features by which they may be distinguished (Campbell & Bunting, 1991). Both focus on the emancipatory goals of research, the use of a variety of methods, the recognition that knowledge is socially constructed, and acknowledgement of the oppressive nature of social structures.

However, critical theorists differ in that gender is not their central concern; they emphasize rationality rather than subjectivity, they write principally for other intellectuals, and power inequalities are maintained within their research teams. Feminist theory, by contrast, places gender centrally within the research, respects and values feelings and experiences, calls for a more equal partnership within research, and claims the importance of making feminist writings accessible to all, not just other intellectuals.

### Research methods in feminist research

Feminist research methods emerge from the epistemological considerations and definitions already discussed. An eclectic stance is generally taken, with researchers wishing to choose methods because they are most appropriate to the topic under consideration, rather than claiming privileged status for any particular method or methods. The advantages of using multiple triangulation are also highlighted by Wilkinson (1986), who writes as a feminist psychologist. However, several further requirements emerge for feminist methods.

Klein (1983) states that intersubjectivity and promoting interaction rather than one-way communication within research is important because:

> 'this will permit the researcher constantly to compare her work with her experiences as a woman and scientist and to share it with those researched, who then will add their opinions to the research, which in turn might change it again.'

Attention has already been drawn also to calls to make relationships within research more equal and less hierarchical. All these elements will increase the vulnerability of the researcher, in the same way that research makes participants vulnerable through disclosing their private experiences and emotions.

These were some of the key points made by Ann Oakley (1981), in a discussion of her experiences of interviewing women who were having babies. Her work was a landmark in writings on research methods and has been influential both within and beyond feminist research. Whilst acknowledging its contribution to the development of feminist research, however, recent writers have made important criticisms of Oakley's paper.

## Interviewing in feminist research: critiques of Oakley's work

Ribbens' (1989) discussion of Oakley's work emerges as a result of her own study as a mother of other women who were also mothers.

Oakley (1981) states that her interviews involved reciprocity between herself and her interviewees in that not only did she ask questions of them, but they asked questions of her too. She found it impossible to adhere to textbook recommendations not to give her own views, and decided to answer interviewees' questions and give information where she could do so based on her own experience.

Ribbens (1989) questions whether this amounted to reciprocity, in that the majority of Oakley's information-giving was of a factual rather than personal nature. For example, she was asked about infant feeding and child development. The extent to which Oakley made herself vulnerable by revealing aspects of herself was therefore very limited, in Ribbens' view.

Questions are also posed about the effect of researcher–interviewee interaction in the communication process. Ribbens (1989) asks whether a researcher's contribution might interrupt an interviewee's train of thought. More importantly, she considers that it may break the 'research contract' in which an interviewee expects to be asked questions and not to receive information about the researcher. This might cause confusing expectations in the minds of interviewees, and lead them to expect a caring response which is not possible within the research relationship because of its limited duration.

Webb (1984) discusses how she shared her own experiences as a gynaecology patient with hysterectomy patients, and how this seemed to have a positive effect and encourage rapport. However, in a more recent interview study with elderly spinsters, sharing personal information about her own health with participants who had had a similar condition did not seem to be welcomed by the women, and Webb ceased to do this once its effect was realized. She speculates that it was the different ages of the spinsters which led them to interpret this sharing differently, whereas younger hysterectomy patients were more similar in age to the interviewer and seemed comfortable with what was said (Webb, 1992).

**One-sided relationship**

Considerations such as these lead Ribbens (1989) to conclude that a one-sided relationship is inevitable, and this view is shared by Wise (1987). Researchers have a different status from those researched. They are usually more highly educated and so are more assertive and articulate. They approach potential participants and ask them to be involved in the project, and thus are in a different and more powerful structural position.

Ribbens (1989) also questions whether forming a relationship with a participant may limit the ability to report adverse findings or to take action when a problem arises, such as uncovering the fact that a woman is abusing her children. Wise (1987), too, draws attention to this point, and says that a feminist approach should not preclude saying negative things about women where this is judged to be appropriate.

These criticisms add up, for Ribbens, to a paradox in which Oakley, at the same time as emphasizing the importance of the presence of the researcher, seems also to be denying it by insisting that power inequalities have been eliminated. Research inevitably involves some degree of inequality and 'exploitation' of informants, because the researcher takes 'their words away to be objectified as an interview transcript'. These risks may be all the greater when multiple interviews take place over an extended period than when they are single events.

Some researchers attempt to overcome problems of inequality by making available to participants data in the form of interview transcripts, research notes and the final report. Some talk about negotiating with participants what will be included and what they may veto. This is the source of another paradox for Ribbens (1989), because there is a:

> 'tension between wanting to get close ... and providing an interpretation ... accounting for women's lives in their own terms and providing a structural analysis'.

**Theoretical discussions**

In other words, researchers aim not simply to describe women's experiences from their own perspectives, but also to develop theoretical discussions of the area of research. In order to do this it is necessary to go beyond individual reports and daily life experiences to examine the influence of wider social structures. Individual participants may only be aware of their own experiences and may have a more limited perspective on social structures than researchers.

Researchers cannot, therefore, restrict themselves to simply reporting the data without analysing them. If participants do not agree with the theoretical interpretation offered, this does not mean it is not a valid one – just as their own and any other person's interpretation is valid for them in the light of the information available to them at the time. In particular, women research participants may not themselves be feminists and therefore might not agree with a feminist interpretation, but the latter may still be valid in its own terms (Ribbens 1989).

With regard to sharing data with participants, it is generally concluded that this should be done to allow them to check the accuracy of the data but that researchers would not necessarily do this with all data, and would reserve the right to make final decisions on what is and is not included in reports (Lather, 1986; Ribbens, 1989).

Ribbens (1989) concludes that:

'All we can attempt is to face up to some of the paradoxes as honestly and explicitly as we can... Ultimately we have to take responsibility for the decisions we make, rather than trying to deny the power that we do have as researchers.'

Wise (1987) similarly calls on feminist researchers to 'acknowledge power where it exists and learn to deal with it wisely as feminists'.

The issue of power within a research relationship and how it can be considered in reporting research will be taken up again below in a discussion of validity in feminist research.

## Feminist ethnography

A number of writers consider that ethnography is particularly appropriate to feminist research (Klein, 1983; Mies, 1983; Reinharz, 1983; Stanley & Wise, 1983). The reason for this is that the participation of the researchers in the everyday lives of those being studied requires replacing the separation of researcher and researched with a relationship which develops over time.

However, for Stacey (1988) these very advantages open up the possibility of greater risks of exploitation, betrayal and abandonment of participants. The process of doing ethnography inevitably involves manipulation, betrayal, inauthenticity and dissimilitude because ethnographers may pretend to be naive when they are not, may conceal from a participant what another has said, and may in other ways misrepresent themselves in order to gain data or check what they have already heard from another source.

A further conflict experienced by Stacey (1988) in her ethnographic study in a community in California, USA, was that on occasions she gained data from people's troubles. For example, she describes how by attending a funeral she benefited from a tragedy.

Finally, the danger that participants in an ethnography will feel abandoned and let down when the researcher leaves the field may be even greater than when the interviewees feel deserted by an interviewer who has entered into a comparatively short relationship with them.

Issues of inequalities of power and ownership of the product of the research are discussed by feminist ethnographers just as they are discussed in relationship to interviewing (Strathern, 1987). Stacey concludes by noting the need to be aware of the possibility that a 'delusion of alliance' will replace the positivist 'delusion of separateness' between ethnographer and participants.

## Reconceptualizing validity and evaluating feminist research

Debates concerning rigour and validity in feminist research take a similar form to those that have taken place over the last few years in relation to qualitative research (see, for example, Morse, 1989). Some qualitative researchers take the view that traditional definitions of concepts such as validity and reliability should be modified and adapted so that they can be readily understood and accepted by those working with 'traditional' definitions used in positivist approaches (Brink, 1991). The latter include referees for grant-giving bodies and academic journals, who are able to control resources for research and gateways to publication.

Others take a contrary position and argue that, since qualitative research operates within a different paradigm, there is no reason to rely on traditional concepts related to rigour and validity. On the contrary, qualitative approaches require new ways of conceptualizing and evaluating rigour (Marshall, 1986). This appears to be the majority view among feminist researchers.

Lather (1986) attempts to 'reconceptualize validity within the context of openly ideological research', which includes critical and feminist research. She offers a set of guidelines by which validity may be evaluated and quotes Cronbach's (1980) reminder that the process of validation is aimed not at seeking support for an interpretation but rather at attempting to falsify it.

Lather (1986) calls for the use of 'data credibility checks' based on a consideration of triangulation, construct validity, face validity and catalytic validity. Triangulation should include the use of multiple sources of data, methods and theoretical schemes and its incorporation within research designs should lead to data trustworthiness in that both 'counterpatterns' and 'convergences' within data can be checked out. Construct validity can be evaluated by means of reflexivity. This means that the researcher systematically reports how decisions were taken at all steps in the research process and how the researcher herself influenced the content and process of the research.

Face validity is assessed by 'member checks', or having research participants 'recycle' the analysis and then refining it according to their reactions. This latter point would not be accepted by all feminist researchers, as was discussed earlier, because the researcher has access to additional perspectives beyond the immediate research and, in order to carry out a structural analysis, would of necessity have to go beyond the immediate data. The notion of catalytic validity relates to the change-promoting aims of feminist research and involves evaluating whether the research has been successful in stimulating change.

Lather (1986) insists that post-modernist approaches, including feminist research, must be based on 'rigor as well as relevance' and that there is no place for 'rampant subjectivity'. It is therefore essential that feminist research is evaluated according to appropriate criteria of the kind she suggests.

## Worthwhileness

Problems of validity are also addressed by Acker *et al.* (1983). They are concerned to evaluate whether feminist research is 'worthwhile' and 'adequate', rather than using the term 'validity'. Worthwhileness for them is similar to Lather's 'catalytic validity' and is concerned with the degree to which the emancipatory goal of the research is achieved. Adequacy is assessed using three criteria which are: whether the voices of participants are heard in research reports; whether the role of the investigator is theorized as well as that of those investigated (which is similar to Lather's emphasis on the need for reflexivity); and whether the analysis reveals the social relations which lie behind the lives of those studied. This last criterion parallels Lather's point about structural analysis.

Hall & Stevens (1991) also prefer the term 'adequacy' to encompass reliability and validity, pointing out that these are closely interconnected. They believe that

'Results are adequate if analytic interpretations fairly and accurately reflect the phenomena that investigators claim to represent.'

Like Lather (1986), they also emphasize the need to check that researchers have not simply verified their own preconceptions.

Evaluating the adequacy of research reports, Hall & Stevens (1991) believe, involves assessing the 'fidelity and authenticity of findings'. This is done by addressing the issues of reflexivity, or whether the researchers have considered:

'their own values, assumptions, characteristics, and motivations to see how they affect theoretic (sic) framework, review of the literature, design, tool construction, data collection, sampling, and interpretation of findings.'

Hall & Stevens (1991) remind us that eliminating 'bias' is impossible and inappropriate in 'passionate scholarship' (Du Bois, 1983) and that a reflexive approach is essential in order to:

> 'make explicit the participation of the researcher in the generation of knowledge, adding to the accuracy and relevance of results.'

### Credibility

Credibility is evaluated by assessing whether participants' experiences have been faithfully represented, and Hall & Stevens' (1991) call for 'member validation' mirrors Lather's point about seeking 'member checks'. Taking this issue further, they also want to assess 'believability' of accounts in the eyes of other feminist researchers. To ensure believability, researchers should ask other researchers to verify the comprehensiveness of literature reviews, the 'effectiveness' of data collection techniques, the 'comprehensibility' of descriptions, the 'inclusivity' of samples, and the logic of the arguments.

The degree of rapport established between researchers and researched, the internal coherence or unity of the report, and the complexity of the analysis should be assessed, according to Hall & Stevens (1991). The latter point relates to how well the complex nature of participants' everyday lives and reality is reflected in the report. Evidence of both consensus and divergence should also be sought, and there should be a discussion of negative cases and alternative explanations.

Feminist research should also demonstrate relevance, that is, appropriateness and significance, to women's concerns and interests. Researchers should show in their reports how they have attempted to reduce power inequalities within research relationships, a point that Hall & Stevens term 'honesty and mutuality'. 'Naming' is required, which parallels earlier calls for women's experiences to be reported in their own words. There should also be evidence to 'relationality', or collaborative working methods with other scholars as well as those being researched.

It is obvious that research outcomes must fit with research definitions and goals, and the three sets of authors quoted suggest how the process of evaluating reports may be tackled. Their recommendations of points to consider when evaluating feminist research reports are summarized in Table 12.1. They use similar concepts and, although their terminology varies slightly, there is clear overlap in the areas they wish to evaluate.

## *Conclusions*

This review of the literature on feminist research has considered definitions, methodology, research methods, and establishing and evaluating rigour. A

**Table 12.1**  Checklists for evaluating feminist research reports summarized from three papers.

| Hall & Stevens (1991) | Acker *et al.* (1983) | Lather (1986) |
|---|---|---|
| Adequacy | Emancipatory goal | Triangulation |
| Reflexivity | Adequacy: | Construct validity |
| Credibility | of reconstruction | Catalytic validity |
| Rapport | in accounting for investigator | Face validity |
| Coherence | in revealing underlying social | |
| Complexity | relations | |
| Consensus | | |
| Relevance | | |
| Honesty and mutuality | | |
| Naming | | |
| Relationality | | |

shorthand definition perhaps could be phrased as 'research *on* women, *by* women, *for* women'. What is distinctive about feminist methodology is its engagement with issues of concern particularly to women and its acceptance of the use of a variety of methods. These methods are used in ways which attempt to reduce power inequalities within research relationships, to report women's experiences in their own terms whilst also attempting a structural analysis of the conditions of their lives, and to include within the analysis the role and influence of researchers themselves.

## Paradoxes and dilemmas

The review has identified a number of paradoxes and dilemmas facing feminist researchers. The way forward must be to continue to acknowledge these issues and to seek ways to resolve them that are consistent with what MacPherson (1983) has called 'a new paradigm for nursing research'.

## *References*

Acker, J., Barry, K. & Esseveld, J. (1983) Objectivity and truth: problems in doing feminist research. *Women's Studies International Forum*, **6**, 423–35.

Adorno, T.W. (1976) Sociology and empirical research. In *Critical Sociology* (ed. P. Connerton), pp. 258–76. Penguin, New York.

Bernhard, L.A. (1984) *Feminist research in nursing research*. Poster session presented at The First International Congress on Women's Health Issues, Halifax, Nova Scotia.

Bernstein, R. (1983) *Beyond Objectivism and Relativism. Science, Hermeneutics and Praxis.* University of Pennsylvania Press, Philadelphia.

Brink, J. (1991) Issues of reliability and validity. In *Qualitative Nursing Research: A Contemporary Dialogue* (ed. J. Morse). Sage, London.

Campbell, J.C. & Bunting, S. (1991) Voices and paradigms: perspectives on critical and feminist theory in nursing. *Advances in Nursing Science*, **13**(3), 1–15.

Cronbach, L. (1980) Validity on parole: can we go straight? *New Directions for Testing and Measurement*, **5**, 99–108.

Du Bois, B. (1983) Passionate scholarship: notes on values, knowing and method in feminist social science. In *Theories of Women's Studies* (eds G. Bowles & R.D. Klein), pp. 105–16. RKP, London.

Evans, M. (1990) The problem of gender for women's studies. *Women's Studies International Forum*, **13**, 457–62.

Habermas, J. (1976) Theory and practice in a scientific society. In *Critical Sociology* (ed. P. Connerton), pp. 330–47. Penguin, New York.

Hall, J.M. & Stevens, P.E. (1991) Rigor in feminist research. *Advances in Nursing Science*, **13**(3), 16–29.

Harding, S. (ed.) (1987) *Feminism and Methodology*. Open University and Indiana University Press, Milton Keynes and Indiana.

Hesse, M. (1980) *Revolution and Reconstruction in the Philosophy of Science*. Indiana University Press, Bloomington, Indiana.

Klein, R.D. (1983) How to do what we want to do: thoughts about feminist methodology. In *Theories of Women's Studies* (eds G. Bowles & R.D. Klein), pp. 88–104. RKP, London.

Kremer, B. (1990) Learning to say no: keeping feminist research for ourselves. *Women's Studies International Forum*, **13**, 463–7.

Lather, P. (1986) Research as praxis. *Harvard Educational Review*, **56**(3), 257–277.

Lather, P. (1988) Feminist perspectives on empowering research methodologies. *Women's Studies International Forum*, **11**(6), 569–81.

McCormack, T. (1981) Good theory or just theory? Toward a feminist philosophy of social science. *Women's Studies International Quarterly*, **4**(1), 1–12.

MacPherson, K.I. (1983) Feminist methods: a new paradigm for nursing research. *Advances in Nursing Science*, **5**(1), 17–25.

Marshall, J. (1986) Exploiting the experience of women managers: towards rigour in qualitative methods. In *Feminist Social Psychology: Developing Theory and Practice* (ed. S. Wilkinson). Open University Press, Milton Keynes.

Mies, M. (1983) Towards a methodology for feminist research. In *Theories of Women's Studies* (eds G. Bowles & R.D. Klein), pp. 117–39. RKP, London.

Morse, J.M. (ed.) (1989) *Qualitative Nursing Research. A Contemporary Dialogue*. Sage, London.

Oakley, A. (1981) Interviewing women: a contradiction in terms. In *Doing Feminist Research* (ed. H. Roberts). RKP, London.

Reinharz, S. (1983) Experiential analysis: a contribution to feminist research. In *Theories of Women's Studies* (eds G. Bowles & R.D. Klein), pp. 162–91. RKP, London.

Ribbens, J. (1989) Interviewing – an 'unnatural situation'? *Women's Studies International Forum*, **12**(6), 579–92.

Stacey, J. (1988) Can there be a feminist ethnography? *Women's Studies International Forum*, **11**, 21–7.

Stanley, L. & Wise, S. (1983) *Breaking Out: Feminist Consciousness and Feminist Research*. RKP, London.

Strathern, M. (1987) An awkward relationship: the case of feminism and anthropology. *Signs*, **12**(2), 276–92.

Webb, C. (1984) Feminist methodology in nursing research. *Journal of Advanced Nursing*, **9**, 249–56.

Webb, C. (1992) The health of single never-married women in old age. *Advances in Nursing and Health*, **11**(6), 3–29.

Wilkinson, S. (ed.) (1986) *Feminist Social Psychology: Developing Theory and Practice*. Open University Press, Milton Keynes.

Wise, S. (1987) A framework for discussing ethical issues in feminist research: a review of the literature. In *Writing Feminist Biography 2: Using Life Histories* (eds V. Griffiths, M. Humm, R. O'Rourke, J. Barsleer, F. Poland & S. Wise), Studies in Sexual Politics No. 19, Department of Sociology, University of Manchester, Manchester.

# Acknowledgements

The chapters in this book are updated papers originally published in the *Journal of Advanced Nursing*. Listed below are references to the original versions.

1 *The outcome and experiences of first pregnancy in relation to the mother's childbirth knowledge: The Finnish Family Competence Study* by Päivi Rautava, Risto Erkkola and Matti Sillanpää: *Journal of Advanced Nursing* (1991) **16**, 1226–32.

2 *Effects of early parent touch on preterm infants' heart rates and arterial oxygen saturation levels* by Lynda Law Harrison, James D. Leeper and Mahnhee Yoon. *Journal of Advanced Nursing* (1990) **15**, 877–85.

3 *Long-term follow-up study of cerebral palsy children and coping behaviour of parents* by Taiko Hirose and Reiko Ueda: *Journal of Advanced Nursing* (1990) **15**, 762–70.

4 *Changing attitudes towards families of hospitalized children from 1935 to 1975: a case study* by Judith Young: *Journal of Advanced Nursing* (1992) **17**, 1422–9.

5 *Qualified nurses' perceptions of the needs of suddenly bereaved family members in the accident and emergency department* by Christopher Tye: *Journal of Advanced Nursing* (1993) **18**, 948–56.

6 *The experience of a community characterized by violence: a challenge for nursing* by Edith Nonhlanhla Madela and Marie Poggenpoel was originally entitled *The experience of a community characterized by violence: implications for nursing: Journal of Advanced Nursing* (1993) **18**, 691–700.

7 *The care and handling of peripheral intravenous cannulae on 60 surgery and internal medicine patients: an observation study* by Anna Lundgren, Lennart Jorfeldt and Anna-Christina Ek: *Journal of Advanced Nursing* (1993) **18**, 963–71.

8 *Patients' experience of technology at the bedside: intravenous infusion control devices* by S. Dianne Pelletier: *Journal of Advanced Nursing* (1992) **17**, 1274–82.

9 *The primary-care nurse's dilemmas: a study of knowledge use and need during telephone consultations* by Toomas Timpka and Elisabeth Arborelius: *Journal of Advanced Nursing* (1990) **15**, 1457–65.

10 *Searching for health needs: the work of health visiting* by Karen I. Chalmers: *Journal of Advanced Nursing* (1993) **18**, 900– 911.

11 *Gay men's perceptions and responses to AIDS* by Grace Getty and Phyllis Stern: *Journal of Advanced Nursing* (1990) **15**, 895–905.

12 *Feminist research: definitions, methodology, methods and evaluation* by Christine Webb: *Journal of Advanced Nursing* (1993) **18**, 416–23.

# Index